LOSE MORE, GAIN LIFE

The Ultimate Guide To Conquering Obesity

Stephen Wood

INTRODUCTION

Obesity is a pathological condition in which excess body fat accumulated, leading to adverse effects on health and life expectancy. It is a chronic disorder with complex interaction between genetic and environmental factors. It characterized by high cholesterol, fatty acid levels; imbalance in metabolic energy; insulin desensitization; lethargy, gallstones; high blood pressure; shortness of breath; emotional and social problems; and excessive adipose mass accumulation with hyperplasia and hypertrophy. Pathological obesity is associated with several secondary commodities like heart disease, type 2 diabetes, breathing difficulties during sleep, cancer, and osteoarthritis't is most commonly caused by a combination of excessive dietary calories, lack of physical activity, and genetic susceptibility. Evidence to support this view is that some obese people eat little yet gain weight due to slow metabolic rate. The primary treatment for obesity are dieting and physical exercise. To supplement this, or in case of failure, anti-obesity drugs may be taken to reduce appetite or inhibit fat absorption. In severe cases, surgery is performed, or an intra-gastric balloon is placed to reduce stomach volume and bowel length, leading to earlier satiation and reduced ability to absorb nutrients from food.

Obesity is one of the leading preventable causes of death worldwide. Currently, beyond 1 billion adults are overweight and at least 300 million of them are clinically obese. Current obesity levels range from below 5% in China, Japan and certain African nations, to over 75% in urban Samoa. Childhood obesity is already epidemic in some areas and on the rise in others. An estimated 17.6 million children under five years. Age are estimated to be overweight worldwide. According to the US Surgeon General, in the USA the number of overweight children has doubled and the number of overweight adolescents has trebled since 1980. The prevalence of obese children aged 6-to-11 years has more than doubled since the 1960s. Obesity prevalence in youths aged 12-17 has increased dramatically from 5% to 13% in boys and from 5% to 9% in girls between 1966-70 and 1988-91 in the USA. The problem is global and increasingly extends into the developing world: In Thailand, the prevalence of obesity in 5-to-12 year olds children rose from 12.2% to 15-6% in just two years. Obesity accounts for 2-6% of total health care costs in several developed countries. The true costs are undoubtedly much greater, r as not all obesity-related conditions are included in the calculations. In the United States obesity is estimated to cause an excess 111,909 to 365,000 death per year, while 1 million (7.7%) of deaths in the European Union are attributed to excess weight.

1. SCALE DEPICTING OVERWEIGHT AND OBESITY

Obesity is usually defined by an indirect measure of body fat, the body mass index(weight (kg)/ (height (m) 2). The international classification of adult weight status was used to classify by body mass index (BMI): (1) underweight (<18.5), (2) normal weight (18.5-24.9), (3) overweight (25.029.9), and (4) obese (>30.0)11. Body mass index does not, however, adequately characterize the distribution of body fat, which is important because excess intra-abdominal fat is an independent predictor of health risk. Waist circumference correlates with visceral fat and indirectly measure central obesity. An increased risk to health is present when waist circumference exceeds 94 cm (37 inches) for men and 80 cm (ca. 31.5 inches.5 inch inches) for women.

CHAPTER ONE

HORMONE AND OBESITY

Obesity is linked to many metabolic disorders and hence the development of obesity can cause changes in metabolic and hormonal conditions, which can result in the storage of excess energy in different forms in the human body. BMI is not considered to be a good estimate of obesity in Asian Indians as they have a characteristic obesity phenotype, with relatively lower BMI but with central obesity. It has been suggested that fat distributed in the abdominal region, particularly visceral fat, is more metabolically important than other fat depots.

Hence, abdominal adiposity assessed using waist circumference is considered to be more appropriate to predict metabolic disorders than generalized adiposity assessed by BMI. The inflammatory response that emerges in the presence of obesity is that it appears to be triggered which reside predominantly in adipose tissue along with other metabolically critical sites which may also be involved during any metabolic diseases. Adipose tissue is now accepted to be an endocrine organ that secretes numerous hormones, growth factors, matrix proteins, enzymes, cytokines, and complement factors that exert multiple effects at both the local and the systemic level.

Secretary factors of adipose tissue and their role in body.

A broad range of protein families, as well as fatty acids and prostaglandins, have been reported to be secreted by adipose tissue. These secreted factors play a role in fat mass regulation and regulation of adipocyte differentiation, vascular and blood flow regulation, lipid and cholesterol metabolism, and immune system function. These factors are not only secreted in mature fat cells but also poorly identified cells present in the stromal–vascular fraction, including macrophages present in extracellular matrix of adipose tissue. Elevated levels of these factors during periods of rapid adipose tissue growth would therefore be expected to increase adipocyte proliferation and differentiation, and potentially program a permanent increase in adipose tissue mass.

Genetics and Obesity

Obesity results from the interaction of environmental factors (overeating or reduction in physical activity or both) and hereditary factors.

Obesity, based on genetics, is a multitude of polymorphisms located in genes and candidate regions throughout the genome that regulate an individual's susceptibility to weight gain in a permissive environment33. Obesity is associated with many genetic syndromes.

There are 20-30 Mendelian disorders in which patients are clinically obese, yet these are additionally distinguished by mental retardation, dysmorphic features, and organ-specific developmental abnormalities. Such cases are referred to as syndromes of obesity. These syndromes arise from discrete genetic defects or chromosomal abnormalities and are both autosomal and X-linked disorders33. The most common disorders known are Prader-Willi syndrome (PWS) and Bardet-Biedl syndrome (BBS), but many others have been reported. A numerous epidemiological study carried out in large and different populations (twins brought up together or separately, adopted children, nuclear families, thus explaining that familiar aggregation for obesity was due to genetic factors rather than environment. The effect of environment on the development of overweight or obesity would be very limited, since the genetic predisposition is present. These results show the importance of identifying families at risk and hence prevent the current and future against childhood obesity.

The genetic factors associated to obesity are depicted as follows:

1) Single mutations contribute to the development of obesity (monogenic obesity).

These forms of obesity are rare, very severe and generally start in childhood.

2) Polygenic obesity, where many genetic variants interact with the environment in common obesity. The risk for common obesity could be due to numerous loci, each with multiple disease predisposing alleles but of low frequency. The genetic study of common

obesity is based on the analysis of variations in genomic DNA (genetic polymorphism or SNP,

Single Nucleotide Polymorphism) situated within or near candidate genes.

Efforts are made to identify candidate genes for obesity, concentrating on adipose tissue. In fat, the regulation of thermogenesis by the sympathetic nervous system is mediated by beta-adrenergic receptors.

In humans, beta-3-adrenergic receptors (?3-AR) are modestly expressed in fat and the adipocytes lining the gastrointestinal tract. Leptin plays an important role in polygenic obesity and was first suggested by linkage studies. A modest reduction of fat-induced leptin secretion may contribute to weight gain. Polymorphisms within the 5? Untranslated region of the human leptin gene were associated with a low leptin level and with resistance to a low-calorie diet.

The peroxisome proliferator-activated receptor-gamma (PPAR?) is a nuclear receptor that plays a key role in adipogenesis and which may lead to efficient energy storage. A Pro12Ala variation in the PPAR? The gene is shown to be associated with improved insulin sensitivity and obesity.

Another approach to identify candidate gene is done by analysis of genome-wide scans to detect chromosomal regions showing linkage with obesity in large collections of nuclear families. To identify the gene variant associated with obesity, chromosomal regions of linkage should first be identified using a dense map of balletic single-nucleotide polymorphisms (SNPs). Recently, in a meta-analysis of genome-wide association studies for WHR adjusted for body mass index, 13 new loci have been identified in or near RSPO3, VEGFA, TBX15-WARS2, NFE2L3, GRB14, DNM3-PIGC, ITPR2-SSPN, LY86, HOXC13, ADAMTS9, ZNRF3-KREMEN1, NISCH-STAB1 and CPEB455. SNPs of adrenoceptors (?1, ?2 and ?3AR), uncoupling proteins (UCPs 1, 2, 3) and PPAR? It were the markers most frequently evaluated in several populations participating in short- or long-term intervention studies. The combined effect of UCP1 and ?3-adrenergic receptor SNPs was found to intensify weight gain in obese individuals during the lifetime. The genetic factors (characterized by the combination of multiple allelic variations), environmental factors (diet, exercise, stress, and hormones), socio-economical factors and the developmental stage of epigenetic events are the useful predictor that can judge the occurrence, development, and maintenance of obesity.

CHAPTER TWO

CAUSES OF OBESITY

It's associated with several related conditions, collectively known as metabolic syndrome. These include high blood pressure, elevated blood sugar and a poor blood lipid profile.

People with metabolic syndrome are at a much higher risk of heart disease and type 2 diabetes, compared to those whose weight is in a normal range.

Over the past decades, much research has focused on the causes of obesity and how it could be prevented or treated.

Obesity and Willpower

Many people seem to think that weight gain and obesity are caused by a lack of willpower.

That's not entirely true. Although weight gain is largely a result of eating behavior and lifestyle, some people are disadvantaged when it comes to controlling their eating habits.

The thing is, overeating is driven by various biological factors like genetics and hormones. Certain people are simply predisposed to gaining weight.

Of course, people can overcome their genetic disadvantages by changing their lifestyle and behavior. Lifestyle changes require willpower, dedication, and perseverance.

Nevertheless, claims that behavior is purely a function of willpower is far too simplistic.

They don't consider all the other factors that ultimately

determine what people do and when they do it.

Here are 10 factors that are leading causes of weight gain, obesity and metabolic disease, many of which have nothing to do with willpower.

1. Genetics

Obesity has a strong genetic component. Children of parents with obesity are much more likely to have obesity than children of lean parents.

That doesn't mean that obesity is completely predetermined. What you eat can have a major effect on which genes are expressed and which are not.

Non-industrialized societies rapidly develop obesity when they start eating a typical Western diet. Their genes didn't change, but the environment and the signals they sent to their genes did.

Put simply, genetic components do affect your susceptibility to gaining weight. Studies on identical twins demonstrate this very well.

2. Engineered Junk Foods

Heavily processed foods are often little more than refined ingredients mixed with additives.

These products are designed to be cheap, last long on the shelf, and taste so incredibly good that they are hard to resist.

By making foods as tasty as possible, food manufacturers are trying to increase sales. But they also promote overeating.

Most processed foods today don't resemble whole foods at all. These are highly engineered products, designed to get people hooked.

3. Food Addiction

Many sugar-sweetened, high-fat junk foods stimulate the reward centers in your brain.

In fact, these foods are frequently compared to commonly abused drugs like alcohol, cocaine, nicotine, and cannabis.

Junk foods can cause addiction in susceptible individuals. These people lose control over their eating behavior, similar to people struggling with alcohol addiction losing control over their drinking behavior.

Addiction is a complex issue that can be very difficult to overcome. When you become addicted to something, you lose your freedom of choice and the biochemistry in your brain starts calling the shots for you.

Some people experience strong food cravings or addiction. This especially applies to sugar-sweetened, high-fat junk foods, which stimulate the reward centers in the brain.

4. Aggressive Marketing

Junk food producers are very aggressive marketers.

Their tactics can get unethical at times, and they sometimes try to market very unhealthy products as healthy foods.

These companies also make misleading claims. What's worse, they target their marketing specifically towards children?

In today's world, children are developing obesity and becoming diabetic and addicted to junk foods long before they're old enough to make informed decisions about these things.

Food producers spend a lot of money marketing junk food, sometimes specifically targeting children, who don't have the knowledge and experience to realize they are being misled.

5. Insulin

Insulin is an essential hormone that regulates energy storage, among other things.

One of its functions is to tell fat cells to store fat and to hold on to the fat they already carry.

The Western diet promotes insulin resistance in many overweight and individuals with obesity. This elevates insulin levels all over the body, causing energy to get stored in fat cells instead of being available for use.

While insulin's role in obesity is controversial, several studies suggest that high insulin levels have a causal role in the development of obesity.

One of the best ways to lower your insulin is to cut back on simple or refined carbohydrates while increasing fiber intake.

This usually leads to an automatic reduction in calorie intake and effortless weight loss — no calorie counting or portion control needed.

6. Certain Medications

Many pharmaceutical drugs can cause weight gain as a side effect.

For example, antidepressants have been linked to modest weight gain over time.

Other examples include diabetes medication and antipsychotics.

These drugs don't decrease your willpower. They alter the function of your body and brain, reducing metabolic rate or increasing appetite.

7. Leptin Resistance

Leptin is another hormone that plays an important role in obesity.

It is produced by fat cells, and its blood levels increase with higher fat mass. For this reason, leptin levels are especially high in people with obesity.

In healthy people, high leptin levels are linked to reduced appetite. When working properly, it should tell your brain how high your fat stores are.

The problem is that leptin isn't working as it should in many people who have obesity because for some reason it cannot cross the blood-brain barrier.

This condition is called leptin resistance and is believed to be a leading factor in the pathogenesis of obesity.

8. Food Availability

Another factor that dramatically influences people's waistline is food availability, which has increased massively in the past few centuries.

Food, especially junk food, is everywhere now. Shops display tempting foods where they are most likely to gain your attention.

Another concern is that junk food is often cheaper than healthy, whole foods, especially in America.

Some people, especially in poorer neighborhoods, don't even have the option of purchasing real foods, like fresh fruit and vegetables.

Convenience stores in these areas only sell sodas, candy and processed, packaged junk foods.

How can it be a matter of choice if there is none?

9. Sugar

Added sugar may be the single worst aspect of the modern diet.

That's because sugar changes the hormones and biochemistry of your body when consumed in excess. This, in turn, contributes to weight gain.

Added sugar is half glucose, half fructose. People get glucose from a variety of foods, including starches, but the majority of fructose comes from added sugar.

Excess fructose_intake may cause insulin resistance and elevated insulin levels. It also doesn't promote satiety in the same way glucose does.

For all these reasons, sugar contributes to increased energy storage and, ultimately, obesity.

10. Misinformation

People all over the world are being misinformed about health and nutrition.

There are many reasons for this, but the problem largely depends on where people get their information from.

Many websites, for example, spread inaccurate or even incorrect information about health and nutrition.

Some news outlets also oversimplify or misinterpret the results of scientific studies, and the results are frequently taken out of context.

Other information may simply be outdated or based on theories that have never been fully proven.

Food companies also play a role. Some promote products, such as weight loss supplements, that do not work.

Weight loss strategies based on false information can hold back your progress. It's important to choose your sources well.

CHAPTER THREE

EFFECT OF OBESITY AND DISEASES CAUSED BY OBESITY

Obesity is a major public health problem which is not only confined to developed countries but it has now become an important public health problem in the world.

High calorie intake in diet due to increased consumption of refined sugars, sweetened beverages, vegetable oils, chunk and fast food and lack of physical activity, absence of playground (open-spaces), sedentary lifestyle all play a role in the development of obesity.

Excess adiposity also known as obesity and excess body weight are associated with increased association with different types of diseases like type 2 diabetes, dyslipidemias, cardiovascular disease, hypertension, and cancer. This review article highlights the pathogenesis, disease association with obesity.

Obesity is a medical condition in which excess body fat has accumulated to the extent that it may have an adverse effect on health, leading to reduced life expectancy and increased health issues. Body mass index (BMI), a measurement which compares weight and height, defines people as overweight (pre-obese) if their BMI is between 25 kg/m2 and 30 kg/m2, and obese when it exceeds 30 kg/m.

BMI is calculated by dividing the subject's mass by the square of his or her height, typically expressed either in metric or US "customary"- unit.

Metric: BMI = kilograms / meters2 US customary and imperial: BMI=lb 703/in

where lb is the subject's weight in pounds and in is the subject's height in inches.

Any BMI of 35 or 40 is severe obesity

A BMI of 35 or 40–44.9 or 49.9 is morbid obesity

A BMI of 45 or 50 is super obesity

BMI	CLASSIFICATION
< 18.5	underweight
18.5–24.9	normal weight
25.0–29.9	overweight
30.0–34.9	class I obesity
35.0–39.9	class II obesity
40.0	class III obesity

CLASSIFICATION OF BODY MASS INDEX (BMI).

2. PATHOGENESIS OF OBESITY

The pathogenesis of obesity is complex and involves humoral and neuronal mechanisms that control appetite and satiety. These stipulations respond to genetic, nutritional, environmental and psychological signals and triggers centers in hypothalamus. The nueruohumoral mechanism that regulate energy balance is divided into three components. The peripheral or afferent systems that create signals from various sites. These include leptin and adiponectin that are produced by fate cells, ghrelin from stomach and peptide from Ileum and colon and insulin from pancreas.

Leptin (meaning thin in Greek Leptos) is a 16kd hormone synthesized by fat cells is the product of ob gene. The leptin receptor (OB-R) is the product of diabetic gene (dg) and belongs to type I cytokine receptor that includes gp130, Granulocyte CSF, IL 6, 2 receptors. Genetically deficient mice in leptin fail to sense fat stores, overeat and gain weight. Adiponectin stimulate fatty acid oxidation, causing a decrease in fat mass. In addition to leptin and adiponectin adipose tissue continuously produces cytokines like TNF, IL 1,6,18, chemokines and steroid hormones that create a chronic subclinical inflammatory state (Asymptomatic) that includes high level of CRP. Ghrelin is produced in the stomach and in the arcuate nucleus of the hypothalamus, and is the only known gut hormone that increases food intake (orexigenic effect). The acute nucleus in the hypothalamus process and integrate signals to generate different signals through two subsets. The first order of neurons include POMC (Promelanocortine) and CART Cocaine and amphetamine regulated transcripts neuron and second order neurons including Neuropeptide Y and AgRP (Agouti related peptide).

The effector system carries signals generated in the second order of neurons of the hypothalamus to control food intake and expenditure. POMT and CART increases energy expenditure and weight loss by producing alpha melanocyte stimulating hormone (MSH) and the activation of melanocortin receptors 3 and 4 (MC3/4) in second order of neurons. NYP/Ag RP neurons promote food intake and weight gain through activation of Y1/5 receptors in secondary neurons.

3. ASSOCIATION OF OBESITY AND DISEASES

Obesity increases the likelihood of various diseases, particularly heart disease, type 2 diabetes, breathing difficulties during sleep, certain types of cancer, and osteoarthritis.

Obesity is most commonly caused by a combination of excessive dietary calories, lack of physical activity, and genetic susceptibility, although a few cases are caused primarily by genes, endocrine disorders, medications or psychiatric illness.

Evidence to support the view that some obese people eat little yet gain weight due to a slow metabolism is limited; on average, obese people have a greater energy expenditure than their thin counterparts due to the energy required to maintain an increased body mass.

There is increased association of obesity and diseases, which are discussed below.

Type1 Diabetes-There is overall evidence for an association between childhood obesity, higher BMI, increased risk of subsequent type1 diabetes.

Type2 diabetes-insulin resistance and hyper insulinaemia. Weight loss associated with improvement. Excess insulin retain Na, expansion of blood volume, production of excess nor epinephrine, smooth muscle proliferation—hallmark of Hypertension.

Osteoarthritis- marked obesity predisposes to degenerative joint disease. Cumulative effect of wear and tear on joint due to obesity, greater the burden of fat, greater the trauma to joints with time.

Gall stone- 6 times more common in obese than non-obese. Increased total cholesterol, increased biliary excretion and cholesterol in bile, cholesterol rich gall stones.

Nonalcoholic steatohepatitis- adolescents and adult who are obese and have type2 diabetes. Fatty change accompanied by inflammation lead to fibrosis.

Dyslipidemia- increased risk of CAD due to hyper TG, Low HDL Syndrome X-distinctive metabolic syndrome-abdominal obesity, insulin resistance, hyper TG, low HDL,HTN,increased risk of CAD.

Thrombosis-increases the risk of is a chromic stroke. Abdominal obesity is associated with increased risk of thrombosis.

Cancer – increased BMI and mortality in cancer esophagus, colon, rectum, liver and NH.

Hypoventilation syndrome- respiratory anomalies, increased sleep both at night and day. Apnic pauses during sleep, polycythaemia and eventually RHF.

4. OBESITY & SYSTEMIC DISEASE ASSOCIATION

GIT-increased gall stone, pancreatitis, Gastrointestinal reflux disease, Nonalcoholic fatty liver disease, abdominal hernia.

Endocrine & Metabolic system-Increased type 2 diabetes, insulin resistance, IGT, dyslipidemia.

Cardiovascular system -increased thromboembolism, Hypertension, Coronary artery disease, Chronic heart failure, Pulmonary hypertension, Asthma.

Female Genital tract/ gynecological -Menstrual abnormality, infertility, carcinoma.

Eye-Cataract

Musculoskeletal system-Osteoarthritis, Gout, Low back pain.

Postoperative-Atelactasis, Pneumonia, Deep vein thrombosis, Pulmonary embolism

Genitourinary-Stress urinary inconvenience.

Neurological-idiopathic inherited.

CHAPTER FOUR

TREATMENT OF OBESITY

To modify the patient's lifestyle, it is necessary to sustain an increase in physical activity and a decrease in food intake. The aim of behavioral therapy is to increase the patient's capacity of self-control.

Based on clinical observations, two hypotheses were put forth to explain overeating:

1) Externality theory – A stimulus control which is conditioned to many external food cues (favorite food, time place, etc.) beside internal stimuli (hunger).

2) Obese eating style- It is a modification of act of eating, where eating quickly by taking large mouthfuls of food and fewer bites. There are also some behavioral techniques of obesity like stimulus control, making patient eat slowly, target setting, self-monitoring (recording weight, meal, and target behavior), social support (family, friends, public health workers).

Pharmacological treatment for patients is assessed at high risk and for those whose dietary and physical activity therapy has not been successful is commonly applied to many other chronic disease states treated by the primary care physician, including cholesterol lowering agents, antihypertensives, and antidiabetic drugs. According to the National Heart, Lung, and Blood Institute (NHLBI) guidelines on the identification, evaluation, and treatment of overweight and obesity in adults and the US Food and Drug Administration (FDA), pharmacotherapy is indicated for: 1) obese patients with a BMI >30 or 2) overweight patients with a BMI >27 and obesity related risk factors or diseases, such as hypertension,

Diabetes, or dyslipidemia.

There involve 5 Potential Strategies for Anti-Obesity Drug Action:

1) **Reducing food intake**: Either amplifies effects of signals/factors that inhibit food intake or block signals/factors that augment food intake.

2) **Acting as appetite suppressants**: Blocking nutrient absorption (especially fat or carbohydrates) in the intestine either by stimulating norepinephrine release (e.g., phentermine, benzphetamine) or block its reuptake into neurons (e.g., mazindol).

3) **Increasing thermogenesis**: Either increase metabolism and dissipate food energy as heat, or increase energy expenditure through the enhancement of physical activity.

4) **Modulating fat metabolism/storage**: Regulate fat synthesis/breakdown by making appropriate adjustments to food intake or energy expenditure.

5) **Modulating the central regulation of body weight**: Either alter

the internal set point or modulate the signals regarding fat stores.

Body weight undergoes a negative feedback control, which involves peripheral and central controllers act as a major role. In this system, the peripheral signals from adipose tissue, muscle, and liver along with hormonal and gastrointestinal signal, provide inferences to the central controllers in the brain, indicating the state of the external and internal environment as they relate to food, metabolic rates, and activity behavior. The central controllers integrate all the signals and transduce these messages into efferent signals governing the behavioral search for the acquisition of food as well as modulating its subsequent deposition into energy storage compartments such as adipose tissue, liver, and muscle by modulating energy expenditure.

Drugs like Orlistat/Xenical,Sibutramine/Meridia,Phentermine/ Adipex, Fastin, Ionamin and others, can be used.

The anti obesity drugs affect appetite, metabolic rate, and inhibit caloric absorption, and generally fall into 3 broad classes:

1) Peripherally acting,

2) centrally acting, and

3) combination (i.e., central and peripheral acting).

Peripherally acting drugs mediate their effects by reducing the calorie absorption in the gastrointestinal system or by affecting metabolic and control systems outside the central nervous system (CNS). Currently, the only peripherally acting anti-obesity drug globally approved for long-term use is orlistat, a lipase inhibitor. Orlistat has been shown to reduce the amount of ingested fat absorption by up to 30% in humans.

Centrally acting drugs act on the CNS by 3 ways: catecholaminergic noradrenaline and

dopamine(e.g., diethylpropion, ethamphetamine, phendimetrazine, and phentermine),5-hydroxytryptamine (5HT) mediated, or combined e.g., sibutramine. Satiety may be regulated through an effect on 5HT, noradrenaline (norepinephrine), or dopamine receptors in the hypothalamus, whereas energy expenditure may be increased directly by thermogenesis and lipolysis or through the stimulation of the sympathetic nervous system. Sibutramine is the only centrally acting drug currently approved for long-term treatment of obesity in adults. Rimonabant (Acomplia, Sanofi-Aventis, Paris, France) is a selective endocannabinoid (CB) 1 receptor antagonist that acts both centrally and peripherally to inhibit food intake and to regulate metabolic functions at diverse peripheral organs, including gut, liver, adipose tissue, and skeletal muscle. Hence, these pharmacological drugs involve the above-mentioned mechanisms and thus regulating the body weight.

CHAPTER FIVE

it's not the complexity of a diet that makes it efficient; it's the careful choice of foods that plays the most important role.

Furthermore, the art of recognizing the nutritional value of different foods and combining them in a way that benefits your body is the key to true weight loss.

A balanced diet is the key to long-term weight loss.

A balanced diet showed to produce a slightly higher weight loss, particularly the loss of fat (Golaye et al., 2010). What's essential to know is that the balanced diet showed to preserve lean body mass. This is essential, as a regular calorie restriction can preserve the fat inside the body, or even slow down fat burning while reducing, or burning, the lean muscle mass. As a result of this, your body doesn't benefit at all. Instead, your metabolism slows down, and the weight loss shown when you step on the scale refers to the loss of muscles. As soon as the diet is over, your body will further pile up calories to compensate for the loss of the lean muscle mass, which consequently results in further weight gain.

The best way to start losing weight long-term is to learn

as much as possible about maintaining a healthy diet. In this spirit, your thoughts and focus while reading this book shouldn't revolve around the number of pounds you want to drop or the dissatisfaction with your figure. It shouldn't revolve around the desired figure either, as this can create a rigid, anxiety-reducing, perfectionist expectation. Instead, your thoughts should focus on discovering what makes a delicious, simple, sustainable, and healthy diet, that will settle all your needs for nutrition without excess fat and toxic food additives.

This means that your criteria for a healthy diet should be:

Variety. Your diet should include a wide range of delicious, natural, healthy, and satisfying foods.

Individuality. Your diet should fit your unique needs and tastes. This applies to both health and personal preference.

Sustainability. Long-term weight loss will require a simple diet. A simple diet is easy to understand, starting from the groceries that will be on your shopping list to daily meal plans and proper food preparation.

Why is a Balanced Diet Important?

A balanced diet was found to be effective for those whose body mass index exceeded 30, and those with endocrine diseases that followed obesity. Essentially, this means that, even if you have hormonal issues alongside obesity, you don't have to overly restrict your diet. Instead, it will be enough to focus on a couple of simple principles and craft a sustainable diet plan that will keep you full and satisfied. You can breathe with ease! A balanced diet that will result in long-term weight loss won't entail giving up your favorite foods, as long as you prepare, serve, and eat them wisely (Golaye et al., 2010).

However, it's also important to note that a balanced lifestyle, alongside a proper diet, played a pivotal role in long-term weight loss. Enough physical activity and sufficient time in the fresh air will be necessary to reap the benefits of your healthy diet. It's ideal to have around one hour of physical activity per day. In addition, attending cognitive-behavioral therapy for dieting can help you establish better self-control when eating, as well as to find better motivation, re-shape your psychological relationship with food, and prevent relapse.

Pay attention to your Menu.

Here's what the participants of most successful studies ate:

Breakfast: Typically, the breakfast consisted of 150g of low-fat skimmed milk, 50g of whole wheat bread, and five grams of butter or margarine. This will come as good news if you like a dose of carby sweetness for breakfast. In addition, this is a simple breakfast one can craft without much fuss. The crucial point is to go for the lean, 0% fat milk and a quality piece of full wheat bread. While it may seem like there's too little to satisfy your morning appetite, keep in mind that complete heat foods are typically more satisfying and satiating than regular bread. Arguably, the same amount of whole-wheat bread will keep you fed a lot longer than the same amount of regular bread. This is because regular bread typically consists of less fiber, and it tends to be airier. This is because the additives inserted in the bread before baking serve to make it light and airy. Expect the whole wheat bread to cost somewhat more than the regular, but it will last longer as smaller amounts will be sufficient to keep you full.

Lunch: For lunch, it's ideal to munch on around 100g of low-fat meat, 150g of vegetables, 60g of either cereal, rice, or pasta, with around 5g of oil. It's important to note that the amounts of oil account for both the oils used to cook the food and those used in dressings and toppings. If you intend to cook multiple dishes for lunch, make sure to distribute the advised amount of oil (5g) across the entire meal. After lunch, your dessert will consist of 100g of fruit.

Snack. After lunch, you can have 180g of low-fat, artificially sweetened yogurt. However, if you find it hard to wait between breakfast and lunch without a snack, you can have your yogurt after breakfast. Keep in mind to skip the afternoon snack, of course.

Dinner: Your evening meal should consist of 100g of either egg or low-fat meat, 60g of pasta, rice, or cereal, and five grams of oil distributed for cooking and seasoning.

Snack. Before bed, you can have 100g of fruit alongside a 50g portion of fresh, low fat (20%) cheese.

As you can see, you can introduce a lot of diversity into a simple, balanced diet. Mainly, you can diversify the types of meats, fruits, and vegetables, as well as ways to prepare the foods. Indeed, five grams of oil per meal is hardly enough to fry even a single omelet. However, you can be creative, and cook numerous dishes misted with oil. After all, this is what this book is for! The simple diet presented in the previous section will be satisfying while introducing no more than 1100 calories per day. In addition, it will include an ideal ratio of macro nutrients needed to secure fat burning instead of muscle burning. According to the previously described plan, you'll eat around 22% of your calories for breakfast, 33% for lunch, 33% for dinner, and 12% for your evening snack.

The first diet plan that was based on seafood included 150g of lean fish three times per week, and the second measured the effects of consuming 150g of fatty fish three times per week. Both of these diets were similar when it came to the composition and ratio of Macro nutrients. Fats took up 30% of the daily calorie intake, while 20% of the diet includes protein. Similar to the balanced diet, carbohydrates took up 50% of the daily calorie intake. The average calorie intake was around 2022 calories for women and 2694 calories for men before the study, while the diet plan given to the participants reduced this intake to 1350 and 1579 calories. On average, men lost around 6.5 kg throughout the course of eight weeks, while women lost 4.2 kg. This study showed that following a diet plan based on seafood results in greater weight loss compared to regular calorie restriction.

These results are explained by the effect of the n-3 fatty acids, particularly in high-quality fish. These acids were found to reduce the fat mass, which is significant to preventing muscle loss in diets.

Another study measured the effects of a regular calorie-restricted diet compared to a restricted balanced diet throughout the course of thirteen weeks. The balanced-deficit diet included a wide range of foods that averaged around 1200 calories per day. The diet plan consisted of 12-15% protein, 25-30% fat, and 50% carbohydrates. This study also noted significantly higher weight loss in participants who followed a balanced diet plan. A reduction in serum leptin was also noted. Leptin is a satiety serum that reduces appetite, driving you to eat smaller amounts of food. This study indicated that the amounts of leptin increased as the diet progressed, helping the participants feel less hungry and more satisfied with their meals (Larsen et al., 2011).

One more important point gained from my research was that a consistent balance in daily eating actually affects the balance between hunger and satiety serums. As you disallow your body to go overly hungry and start starving, on a physiological level, it begins to trust that there's no reason for triggering hunger because you'll care for your needs in time. Once I learned this, it became clear that the next step is to craft an inclusive diet that simply must keep me full. This will be your task as well, and I'll show you how to do it in the following sections.

2. IDEALS FOR BALANCE DIET MEAL

As you already know, a balanced diet requires dividing the intake of macro nutrients to about 50% carbohydrates and 25/30% carbs and protein. A moderate calorie reduction of up to 30% should yield long-term weight loss. But, how to put this in motion? How does one really create a balanced meal?

It's not always easy to determine what a "balanced" meal is. The key to a balanced reduction diet is to reduce, or control, portion sizes, while increasing the variety of foods. In addition, a successful diet will require cutting out processed foods, artificial sugars, and alcohol from your daily routine. More than that, it will require useful ideas for food preparation.

The simplicity of the diet plays a crucial role in weight loss, as it is close to impossible to emulate the conditions of study-tailored diets without medical monitoring. You won't be able to evaluate the composition of your meals under a microscope or detect the exact calorie count. For this reason, sufficient knowledge of foods and their distribution of macronutrients will be essential.

When it comes to the distribution of macronutrients in your diet, it's vital to spread your proteins, carbs, and fats evenly throughout the day. Ideally, you won't mix carbs and fats within a single meal, as this will spike your post-meal insulin levels. This could cause your existing fat supplies to further increase.

However, most studies highlight that long-term weight loss requires a permanent change in lifestyle. Mainly, this applies to physical activity and eating patterns. What is an eating pattern? Most of us have steady dietary habits, out of which many aren't good. We eat on the go, out of boredom, or simply to avoid throwing away food. One of the good ways to evaluate dietary habits is to keep a food journal. It's recommended to track your eating over the course of one week, noting everything you eat and drink throughout the day. This includes sweets, snacks, sodas, alcohol, and pretty much everything you consume.

Moreover, make sure to review your fridge, and figure out what mainly makes for your daily diet. It's also important to think about the variety of foods you eat and your meal habits. Do you eat in a rush, on the go, or sit down to have a small meal? What are your criteria for choosing foods? Do you do it based on taste, or do you think about health as well?

In addition to that, it's also indispensable to think about your portion sizes. Do you think about sufficient amounts of food when eating, or you fill your plate without thinking through it?

Your food journal should also contain the times you decide to eat. Do you have a steady eating schedule, or do you eat whenever you have the time? Perhaps, you only eat once per day? Do you have regular meals, or do you skip breakfast or lunch?

If you want to lose weight and feel well-nourished, you'll have to figure out a way to change your eating patterns. Since "balance" can mean different things to different people, defining it is necessary so that you can understand how to actually change your diet.

The majority of popular diets revolve around counting macro nutrients and defining the right ratio of fats, protein, and carbohydrates for weight loss. Some of these diets are truly effective, while others lead to nothing more than a short-term weight loss of a couple of pounds, followed by the subsequent weight gain. Often, carbohydrates get scapegoated in the curious case of weight gain, after which they're banished and replaced by liquids, supplements, or an abundant amount of protein. Alas, this sort of imbalance in eating deprives you of an important energy source. As you learned, the problem in weight gain isn't in carbohydrates, but rather the way they're consumed. Mainly, the highest concentration of food is consumed in the evening when the physical activity is close to none. For that reason, a balanced diet doesn't banish carbohydrates. Instead, it uses them wisely to obtain a source of energy early and then favors protein and fiber for the body to wind down in the evening.

In fact, a balanced diet doesn't only account for the ratio of macro nutrients. Instead, it encompasses your whole relationship with food, involving the mealtimes, amounts, and variety of different foods, all well-organized to give you exactly what you need in the particular time of the day. When thinking about a balanced diet, care for the times, amounts, and varieties you eat much as you would about calorie count and macro nutrient ratio. After all, the research I presented you with does confirm that lifestyle changes and adherence to the program play an important role as the calorie count.

Foods that are rich in carbohydrates are best designed to supply you with enough energy throughout the afternoon. However, you would rather not exaggerate the number of carbohydrates because they can make you sleepy. The ideal choice and amounts of healthy carbs will give you enough blood sugar, but without the consequent feeling of sluggishness.

This includes whole grains that are high in fiber. For this, you can choose barley, and other whole grains like wheat, or rice.

CHAPTER SIX

REASONS WHY YOU NEED TO LOSE WEIGHT

Your weight may impact how you feel about yourself and even how others see you, yet self-perception isn't the main explanation you ought to leave on a weight-misfortune venture.

Truth be told, for the individuals who are overweight or hefty, shedding pounds really conveys incalculable advantages past glancing incredible in your new garments.

Eventually, being overweight has a great deal of symptoms, from seemingly insignificant details like back torment to progressively genuine results like being bound to create type 2 diabetes. Other than limiting these health issues, there are additionally countless little-known advantages that accompany a trimmer figure. Peruse on to find a few experiences into how your body and lifestyle can change after pounds. You'll have even more motivation to fight the lump, as analysts have discovered that when you think of solid inspirations to lose weight before leaving on your excursion, you lose more weight than the individuals who are less propelled!

17 reasons why you need weight lost.

1. Gain Confidence

That feeling you experience after you step on the scale and see you're 5 pounds (2.27 kilogram) lighter isn't simply alleviation. It's likewise the trust in your achievement and in realizing you've assumed responsibility for your life to improve things— and you have the outcomes to demonstrate it. One Reddit client, superfluous1, who lose 140 pounds went to the acknowledgment that he wasn't an inalienably languid individual: I've been overweight for the vast majority of my life, and it generally felt like an ethical coming up short. I presently understand that being fat makes you sluggish. It damages to stroll, to remain, to live—no big surprise, all I needed to do was plunk down or rest, He finishes up, "Being apathetic didn't make me fat—I was lethargic because I was fat." But if you are drowsy, attempt these sluggish approaches to lose weight!

2. People Will Be Nicer To You

If it were up to us, it wouldn't be this way. In any case, truth is, our public often oppresses overweight individuals, regardless of whether that implies they'll gather less consideration from healthcare suppliers or get increasingly negative remarks from peers. (It's scientifically demonstrated!) But, after you've shed pounds, you'll begin to see things change. Individuals who once overlooked you may welcome you with a grin or significantly offer to keep the door open for you. "I have shed 120 pounds now, and individuals treat me so much differently," composes Fat Secret message board client girly girl at heart. Client jkessler9508 concurs: "Dismal, however obvious… it appears everybody is more pleasant to you [after you lose weight.]"

3. You'll Breathe Better

Thinning down has been appeared to improve oxygen productivity, so you likely won't get as winded going up the stairs or taking care of your little ones.

4. YOU MAY BE ABLE TO TOSS YOUR MEDS

There are notable long haul advantages of weight misfortune, yet in any event, losing a little weight presently can improve your life by reducing indications of ebb and flow sicknesses right away! That implies you may have the option to take lower portions of your present prescriptions or quit taking certain medications out-and-out. (One more approach to set aside cash!) Check in with your primary care physician and see what kinds of changes the person in question figures the slimmer you may profit by.

5. Your Cancer Risk Will Decrease

The vast majority realize that smoking and sunning can up your disease hazard, however hardly any individuals understand that weight is connected to malignant growth as well. (Specialists accept that a similar irritation that causes weight gain causes DNA-harm and the subsequent infections.) That's the awful news. The uplifting news, in any case, is that you can diminish levels of aggravation by losing only five percent of your body weight, as indicated by a Cancer Research investigation of postmenopausal ladies.

6. Reduction in Snoring

Incredible for you—and your accomplice! Two rest issues, rest apnea and wheezing, are often brought about by overabundance of weight around the neck. Therefore, both annoying conditions can disappear nearby a weight loss of only 5 percent, as per a survey distributed in Sleep.

7. Your Wallet Will Be Thicker

Weight gain costs us a ton of cash—and we're not simply discussing shirts and jeans tore by scraping or popped skirt catches. The individuals who check in at a healthy weight spend a bewildering 42 percent less money on hospital expenses and health costs than their overweight friends, as per a Health Affairs report. Sure health care is a serious enormous gouge in your budgetary future, yet in addition consider all that cash you'll spare by cooking at home, instead opting out at cafés, leaving the soft drink on the rack, and saying "no" to that third adjust of liquor.

8.You Eat New Foods

Eating ineffectively sure gets exhausting. It's only plenty of pizza cuts, burgers, and flame broiled cheeses. Then again, when you're preparing home-prepared meals, you'll figure out how to attempt new plans, acclimate yourself with the supermarket, and even look at the rancher's market! Get your staple rundown out and begin by picking a formula from our rundown of the zero tummy plans.

9. You'll Try New Activities

With such additional weight, you may have been restricted in what sorts of activities, exercises, or even excursions you could go on. With a trimmer edge, anticipate taking part in open air exercises you were never ready to take part in like climbing, kayaking, skiing, mountain biking, surfing, or rock ascending. You can even get the entire family included!

10. YOU MAY BE ABLE TO TOSS YOUR MEDS

There are notable long haul advantages of weight misfortune, yet in any event, losing a little weight presently can improve your life by reducing indications of ebb and flow sicknesses right away! That implies you may have the option to take lower portions of your present prescriptions or quit taking certain medications out-and-out, more approach to set aside cash! Check in with your primary care physician and see what kinds of changes the person in question figures the slimmer you may profit by.

11. You'll Make New Friends.

Grinding away alone isn't in every case simple. When you pursue wellness classes, individual instructional courses, cooking classes, or training camps, you'll be more than likely to meet individuals experiencing a comparable excursion en route. In any event, finding an exercise pal or a collaborator to keep you legitimate is an incredible procedure for weight misfortune. Welcome somebody from your turn class over to make one of these healthy chicken plans.

12.You'll Live Longer

You may have just speculated, yet a less fatty you liken to a diminished danger of malady, and in this way, a more drawn out life. We realize you needn't bother with a lot of confirmation, yet you probably won't need to know the degree of stoutness has an effect on your lifespan; A meta-examination of 20 investigations, distributed in PLOS Medicine, found that extraordinary weight may abbreviate your life anticipation as long as 14 years! The individuals who are overweight or fat who shed 3 percent of their weight won't just observe health benefits yet may likewise broaden their life by two years, as per the British National Institute for Health and Care Excellence.

13. YOUR SEX DRIVE WILL IMPROVE

Desert, the room blues. As your BMI falls, you'll all the more effectively become stimulated. It's everything because of the ascent in testosterone levels that accompanies burning endlessly muscle versus fat. In an investigation distributed in the Journal of Clinical Endocrinology and Metabolism, heavier men had T-levels practically identical to old gentlemen about an entire decade more seasoned. Different investigations have discovered that ladies with stomach fat amassing have raised discharges of cortisol, a pressure hormone. More cortisol—and in this manner higher feelings of anxiety—was found to meddle with sexual excitement. Other than what's new with your body within, losing that overhang may permit you to feel less hesitant naked, which can expand your longing to get it on as well.

… And You'll Enjoy It More!

14. Your Memory May Improve

Try not to accuse a dependence for your wireless as the explanation that you can't recall telephone numbers or names any longer. Your meandering personality may likewise be an aftereffect of hauling around additional weight. In one investigation, ladies performed better on memory tests following shedding pounds than they did before dropping the pounds. Why? The mind checks uncovered that once the ladies shed pounds, there was greater action while they were shaping recollections and less movement during memory proposed, that carrying around additional L-B's may make it increasingly difficult for the cerebrum to work effectively. Different examinations have discovered that the principle segment in pop and other improved nourishment—fructose—disturbs the production of new pathways between synapses that happens when we learn or experience something new. Specialists have discovered that cut the sweet stuff from your eating routine and increasing your admission of these omega-3 superfoods during your weight misfortune can battle this cerebrum channel.

15. You Won't Constantly Seek Food

While crash health food nuts often feel hungrier after thinning down in gratitude to the body's endurance reaction to build hunger hormones and moderate digestion when it's famished, that isn't the situation for everybody. The individuals who follow expanded plans that join healthy nourishment pressed with satiety-boosting supplements like protein and fiber—like the Zero Belly Diet—often report less stomach thunders. In addition, these healthy eating regimens regularly cut out immediately processed nourishment that spike your glucose, cautioning your body it's ravenous not long after eating. Look at what else adds to those treat desires in our selective story—reasons why you're constantly eager.

16. You Won't Sweat As Much

Does it ever feel like you're in a sauna when it's only 70 degrees? This is because fat protects the body and raises center temperature, causing you to feel hotter than the individuals who are slimmer. For a similar explanation, overweight people will in general perspiration more. Drop the overhang and you won't need to walk directly to the washroom to towel off after strolling anyplace.

17. Your Job May Seem Easier

Having a slimmer body prompts a more astute cerebrum? Maybe! As per an investigation distributed in the diary Frontier's in Nutrition, men who haul around additional pounds have more unfortunate intellectual abilities than their trimmer partners.

CHAPTER SEVEN

*29 healthy, weight-loss-friendly
snacks to add to your diet.*

Snacking refers to the intake of foods during the day apart from your main meals. Snacks typically consist of smaller food portions distributed between meals.

While research on whether snacking aids weight loss is mixed, some evidence suggests that increasing your meal frequency through snacking may help manage hunger and improve blood sugar regulation.

Additionally, snacking can help you increase your intake of nutrient-rich foods like fruits and vegetables — and most people are not eating enough produce.

Aim for snacks that include protein, fiber, and healthy fats, which help keep you full throughout the day and make healthy choices at your next meal.

By planning ahead and focusing on nutrient-rich foods, snacks may support your weight management goals by managing hunger and keeping you satisfied between meals.

While no one snack will lead to weight loss, these snacks may help promote weight loss as part of an overall healthy eating pattern.

Here are 29 healthy, weight-loss-friendly snacks to add to your diet.

1. Mixed nuts

Nuts are an ideal nutritious snack, providing the perfect balance of healthy fats, protein, and fiber.

Aside from being tasty, they're linked to numerous health benefits and very filling. Studies also suggest that despite their higher calorie and fat content, eating nuts in moderation may help you lose weight.

There are plenty of nuts you can choose from, including walnuts, almonds, Brazil nuts, hazelnuts, pine nuts, macadamia nuts, cashews, and pistachios.

Because they don't require refrigeration, they're a great choice for snacking on the go. Be mindful of your portion size, and aim to stick to about 1 ounce or 1/4 cup.

2. Red bell pepper with guacamole

The combo of red bell peppers and guac gives you plenty of nutrients that help keep you feeling full for hours.

Although all bell peppers are nutritious, red varieties are particularly high in antioxidants. On the other hand, guacamole is a rich source of healthy fats, fiber, vitamins A, B, and C, and minerals like phosphorus and potassium.

Pairing 1 large red bell pepper with 3 ounces (85 grams) of guacamole combines the best of both foods while keeping this snack's calorie count under 200.

3. Greek yogurt and mixed berries

Plain Greek yogurt and berries make a delicious, nutrient-dense snack.

Greek yogurt is high in protein, and berries are one of the best sources of antioxidants around.

Add a mixture of differently colored berries to your yogurt to get an array of nutrients — and a mix of their sweet and tart flavors.

4. Apple slices with peanut butter

Apples and peanut butter are a match made in heaven — both nutritionally and flavor-wise.

On one hand, apples are a fiber-rich fruit. On the other hand, peanuts provide healthy fats, plant-based protein, and fiber — almost all telling nutrients you should look for in a snack.

By combining apples with peanut butter, you'll enjoy a crisp and creamy snack. Try adding a sprinkle of cinnamon for an added flavor boost.

Note that many store-bought peanut butter brands contain added sugars and oils. Check the ingredient list and choose one that only contains peanuts and salt.

5. Cottage cheese and fruit

Cottage cheese is high in filling protein, boasting 24 grams in just 1 cup (0.24 liters).

Pairing cottage cheese with fruit complements the cheese's protein and fat content with the fruit's fiber, resulting in a sweet, creamy, and filling snack.

The combination is perfect when combining the cheese with tropical fruits such as pineapple, papaya, or watermelon.

6. Celery sticks with cream cheese

Celery sticks with cream cheese are a class low-carb snack that can help keep you feeling full.

This duo will have you enjoying a fiber-packed snack that combines a crunchy texture from the celery with creaminess from the cheese. Try celery sticks with peanut butter or almond butter for another crunchy and creamy combo.

Snacking on 5 small celery sticks with about 1 ounce (30 grams) of cream cheese provides roughly 100 calories.

7. Kale chips

Kale_is incredibly healthy, as it's loaded with fiber and antioxidants like beta-carotene, lutein, and zeaxanthin.

It's also a good source of minerals, such as calcium and phosphorus. It has a lower level of oxalic acid, an anti-nutrient that impairs calcium absorption, than many other leafy greens.

Pairing kale with olive oil not only makes more delicious and crispy chips, but also a more balanced and filling snack.

This easy recipe for kale chips provides about 150 calories:

Kale chips

Ingredients:

- 1 cup (20 grams) of bite-sized kale leaves
- 1 tablespoon (15 mL) of olive oil
- 1/4 teaspoons (1.5 grams) of salt

Directions:

Mix all ingredients in a bowl. Place kale pieces on a parchment-lined baking sheet and bake at 350 °F (ca. 177 °C) for 10–15 minutes, until crispy and starting to slightly brown. Watch them closely, as they can easily burn.

8. Dark chocolate and almonds

Dark chocolate_and almonds are a fantastic pair. The rich chocolate flavor paired with the crunchy nuts is a powerful flavor and health duo.

Dark chocolate contains antioxidants, and almonds_are a rich source of healthy fats.

The two make a great combo for a heart-healthy, satisfying, and portable snack. Try a couple of teaspoons of dark chocolate chips or a square of dark chocolate with a handful of nuts.

9. Cucumber slices with hummus

Cucumber's fresh flavor and crunchy texture go very well with the rich creaminess of hummus.

Hummus is typically made from chickpeas, tahini, olive oil, and garlic. Thus, it provides a mix of plant-based protein, fiber, and heart-healthy fats.

Enjoying 1 cup (104 grams) of sliced cucumbers dipped in 2 tablespoons (34 grams) of hummus will help keep you full for under 100 calories.

You can also pair them with some whole grain crackers or pretzel sticks for a heartier snack.

10. A piece of fruit

Healthy snacks don't need to be complicated. Just a single piece of fruit can be incredibly satisfying.

Portable, easy-to-eat fruits include bananas, apples, pears, grapes, grapefruit, and oranges.

Fruit contains fiber and minerals and makes a great small snack. To make it more satisfying, pair your fruit with nuts or yogurt.

11. Cherry tomatoes with mozzarella

Tomatoes and mozzarella cheese are a nutritious and yummy way to add more veggies to your diet.

Mix tomatoes_with mozzarella, balsamic vinegar, and a drizzle of olive oil for a snack with protein, fiber, and healthy fats.

This tasty and fresh snack can also double as a side salad for your next meal.

12. Chia pudding

Chia seeds are tiny nutritional powerhouses loaded with fiber, omega-3 fatty acids, and plant-based protein.

Although they don't have much flavor, chia seeds_take on a jelly-like consistency when soaked in liquid, making them a great ingredient for puddings.

Try this simple recipe for a healthy snack to enjoy at home or on the go:

Chia seed pudding

Ingredients:

- 1 tablespoon (15 grams) of chia seeds
- 1/3 cup (709.76 cm^3) of a dairy or nondairy milk of your choice
- 1/2 tablespoon (8 grams) of cocoa powder or peanut butter for flavor
- 1/2 cup (75 grams) of mixed berries
- 1–2 teaspoons sweetener, like maple syrup or honey, if desired

Directions:

Combine chia seeds and a liquid of your choice in a small bowl or jar. Cover the jar and refrigerate it for at least 30 minutes. Stir in cocoa powder or peanut butter and sweetener, and top it with the berries.

13. Hard-boiled eggs

Eggs are one of the healthiest and most weight-loss-friendly food you can eat. They are incredibly filling, thanks to their protein content.

Although their high cholesterol levels gave them a bad reputation for years, recent studies suggest that moderate egg intake — defined as 3–4 eggs per week — may benefit arterial stiffness, a risk factor for heart disease.

Additionally, hard-boiled eggs are a convenient way to enjoy a high-protein snack while on the go. Keep the yolk to get important nutrients like vitamin D and choline.

14. Baby carrots with blue cheese dressing

Baby carrots with blue cheese dressing are the perfect snack for when you crave something savory.

In addition, it's a good idea to pair carrots with a creamy salad dressing or dip, as aside from keeping you fuller for longer, fat increases your absorption of carrot's fat-soluble micronutrients, such as carotenoids.

While blue cheese dressing on its own isn't nutrient-rich, it may help you eat more carrots (or other veggies).

A 3.5-ounce (100-gram) serving of baby carrots with 2 tablespoons (30 grams) of blue cheese dressing serves as a light snack, containing about 180 calories.

15. Cheese with crackers or fruit

Cheese is a delicious, high-protein food that's filling enough to be a snack on its own. However, pairing it with whole grain crackers or a piece of fruit adds some fiber to your snack.

Go with the cheese you're desiring or try mozzarella, ricotta, or feta. Cheese delivers protein and calcium, but the amounts of those nutrients vary slightly depending on the type you choose.

You could spread a bit of cheese on your favorite whole grain crackers or opt for string cheese with a piece of fruit for a convenient on-the-go option.

16. Beef jerky or beef sticks

Beef jerky_or beef sticks make excellent high protein, portable snacks. That said, depending on the brand and flavoring, some are higher in added sugar and sodium.

Look for jerky with as few added ingredients as possible. Although all jerky can be high in sodium, the flavored jerky tends to be higher in sodium, so check the nutrition facts panel to find an option without too much salt.

Look for jerky with less than 300 mg of sodium per serving, which accounts for 13% of the Daily Value (DV) of the mineral.

Most beef jerkins and sticks contain about 7 grams of protein per ounce (28 grams).

17. Protein smoothie

A protein smoothie can be a filling snack for when you need something substantial until your next meal.

They're an easy and convenient way to increase your protein intake. You can add just about any other ingredient to the mix, from fruits and veggies to healthy fats like avocado, nut butter, or chia seeds, for a nutrient-rich snack.

While you can choose from a wide array of protein powders to find the one that suits you best, you can also try Greek yogurt or silken tofu to boost the protein content of your smoothie.

18. Whole wheat toast with canned fish

Canned fish, such as canned salmon, sardines, and tuna, may not be the first food that comes to mind when you think of snacks, but it's a fantastic option that requires no refrigeration.

Plus, salmon_and sardines are incredibly high in omega-3 fatty acids, which decrease your risk of heart disease, inflammation, and other health problems.

Topping a piece of whole wheat toast with canned fish will give you a highly nutritious snack that will leave you feeling full until your next meal. For something smaller, try a few whole grain crackers with tuna or salmon.

19. Edamame

Edamame is a dish of steamed unripened soybeans that makes a great snack for anyone following a vegan or vegetarian diet.

It's a fiber-rich food that's considered a complete, plant-based protein source.

One cup (155 grams) of edamame_provides around 18 grams of protein and 13 grams of carbs, 8 of which come from fiber.

20. Oatmeal

Oatmeal is a truly versatile snack that you can enjoy hot or cold — at home or on the go. Just whip up a slightly smaller portion of oats than you might for a meal.

Oats are a nutritious whole grain that provides a good amount of fiber and higher protein content compared with other cereals.

What's more, you can satisfy your sweet tooth with oatmeal topped with fruit, cinnamon, cocoa powder, and chocolate chips, or go for a savory version by adding eggs, avocado, and veggies like mushrooms or tomatoes.

21. Pear slices with ricotta cheese

Pear slices and ricotta cheese make a satisfying snack with a sweet taste and creamy texture, and it provides fiber and protein.

22. Homemade trail mix

Make a trail mix by combining dried fruit and nuts for fiber, protein, and healthy fats. Choose fruits without added sugar and get creative with flavors. Try dried mango with cashews, dried apples with almonds, and dried cherries with peanuts.

While homemade trail mix is perfect for on-the-go snacking, stick to a modest portion size, as dried fruit and nuts are calorie-dense.

23. Turkey roll-ups

Turkey roll-ups are delicious and nutritious.

Turkey contains high-quality protein, which helps you feel satisfied and is linked to beneficial effects on weight management.

Try rolling up a slice of turkey with a slice of cheese and some vegetables for added crunch and nutrients.

24. Olives with feta cheese

Olives are one of the nutritious staples of the Mediterranean diet.

They're very high in heart-healthy monounsaturated fats and provide powerful antioxidants.

Combine olives with feta cheese for a Greek-inspired snack that's rich in protein and healthy fats. You could eat them by themselves or serve them over whole wheat bread to complete your snack with some complex carbs.

25. Spicy avocado

Avocados are among the most nutritious and satisfying foods due to their high fat and fiber content.

Sprinkle half of a medium avocado with salt and a dash of cayenne pepper for a savory, filling snack under 120 calories.

26. Popcorn

But think air-popped popcorn — not the movie-theater kind doused in butter and salt.

Popcorn delivers filling fiber and less than 100 calories in a generous 3-cup serving.

Add flavor with a bit of olive oil, Parmesan cheese, or nutritional yeast.

27. Roasted chickpeas

Roasting chickpeas helps turn them into a crunchy and delightful snack.

Chickpeas are a source of fiber and plant-based protein.

You can make your own or look for roasted chickpeas in the snack section of your grocery store.

28. Cantaloupe slices wrapped in prosciutto

Cantaloupe is a nutritious, delicious fruit delivering fiber and vitamins A and C.

Combining cantaloupe with prosciutto (dry-cured ham) creates a balanced, sweet-and-salty snack.

Try wrapping 4 medium cantaloupe wedges (276 grams) with a thin slice of prosciutto each for a snack under 180 calories.

29. Last night's leftovers

One great way of taking advantage of your leftovers from a nutritious lunch or dinner is by having them as a snack.

By getting a smaller portion of a previous meal, you'll enjoy a complete and balanced snack in seconds.

Just make sure to store your leftovers in the refrigerator to keep them from spoiling quickly.

CHAPTER EIGHT

No matter what your weight loss goals are, losing weight can feel impossible at times.

However, shedding a few pounds doesn't have to involve a complete overhaul of your current diet and lifestyle.

In fact, making a few small changes to your morning routine can help you lose weight and keep it off.

This article lists 10 simple morning habits to incorporate into your regimen to aid your weight loss efforts.

1. Eat a High-Protein Breakfast

There's a good reason breakfast is considered the most important meal of the day.

What you eat for breakfast can set the course for your entire day. It determines if you'll feel full and satisfied until lunch, or if you'll be heading to the vending machine before your mid-morning snack.

Eating a high-protein breakfast may help cut cravings and aid in weight loss.

In one study in 20 adolescent girls, eating a high-protein breakfast reduced post-meal cravings more effectively than a normal-protein breakfast.

Another small study showed that eating a high-protein breakfast was associated with less fat gain and reduced daily intake and hunger, compared to a normal-protein breakfast.

Protein_may also aid weight loss by decreasing levels of ghrelin, the "hunger hormone" that is responsible for increasing appetite.

In fact, one study in 15 men found that a high-protein breakfast suppressed ghrelin secretion more effectively than a high-carb breakfast.

To help get your day off to a good start, consider protein sources like eggs, Greek yogurt, cottage cheese, nuts, and chia seeds.

2. Drink Plenty of Water

Starting your morning with a glass or two of water is an easy way to enhance weight loss.

Water can help increase your energy expenditure, or the number of calories your body burns, for at least 60 minutes.

In one small study, drinking 16.9 fluid ounces (0.5 l) of water led to a 30% increase in metabolic rate, on average.

Another study found that overweight women who increased their water intake to over 34 ounces (1.29 kg) (one liter) per day lost an extra 4.4 pounds (2 kg) over one year, without making any other changes in their diet or exercise routine.

What's more, drinking water may reduce appetite and food intake in some individuals.

One study in 24 older adults showed that drinking 16.9 fluid ounces (0.5 l) of water reduced the number of calories consumed at breakfast by 13%.

In fact, most studies on the topic have shown that drinking 34–68 ounces (1–2 liters) of water per day can aid in weight loss.

Starting your morning with water and staying well hydrated throughout the day is a great way to boost weight loss with minimal effort.

Increasing your water intake has been associated with an increase in weight loss and energy expenditure, as well as a decrease in appetite and food intake.

3. Weigh Yourself

Stepping on the scale and weighing yourself each morning can be an effective method to increase motivation and improve self-control.

Several studies have associated weighing yourself daily_with greater weight loss.

For instance, a study in 47 people found that those who weighed themselves daily lost about 13 pounds (ca. 6 kg) more over six months than those who weighed themselves less often.

Another study reported that adults who weighed themselves daily lost an average of 9.7 pounds (4.4 kg) over a two-year period, while those who weighed themselves once a month gained 4.6 pounds (2.1 kg).

Weighing yourself every morning can also help foster healthy habits and behaviors that may promote weight loss.

In one large study, frequent self-weighing was associated with improved restraint. Furthermore, those who stopped weighing themselves frequently were more likely to report increased calorie intake and decreased self-discipline.

For best results, weigh yourself right when you wake up. Do so after using the bathroom and before you eat or drink anything.

Additionally, remember that your weight may fluctuate daily and can be influenced by a variety of factors. Focus on the big picture and look for overall weight loss trends, rather than getting fixated on small day-to-day changes.

Studies have found that daily self-weighing may be associated with more weight loss and increased restraint.

4. Get Some Sun

Opening the curtains to let in some sunlight or spending a few extra minutes outside each morning can help kick-start your weight loss.

One small study found that exposure to even moderate levels of light at certain times of the day can have an influence on weight.

Moreover, an animal study found that exposure to ultraviolet radiation helped suppress weight gain in mice fed a high-fat diet.

Exposure to sunlight is also the best way to meet your vitamin D_needs. Some studies have found that meeting your vitamin D requirements can aid in weight loss and even prevent weight gain.

In one study, 218 overweight and obese women took either vitamin D supplements or a placebo for one year. At the end of the study, those who met their vitamin D requirement lost an average of 7 pounds (3.18 kg) more than those with inadequate vitamin D blood levels.

Another study followed 4,659 older women for four years and found that higher levels of vitamin D were linked to less weight gain.

The amount of sun exposure you require can vary based on your skin type, the season, and your location. However, letting in some sunlight or sitting outside for 10–15 minutes each morning may have a beneficial effect on weight loss.

Sun exposure may have an influence on weight. Sunlight can also help you meet your vitamin D needs, which may help increase weight loss and prevent weight gain.

5. PRACTICE MINDFULNESS

Mindfulness is a practice that involves fully focusing on the present moment and bringing awareness to your thoughts and feelings.

The practice has been shown to enhance weight loss and promote healthy eating habits.

For example, an analysis of 19 studies found that mindfulness-based interventions increased weight loss and reduced obesity-related eating behaviors.

Another review had similar findings, noting that mindfulness training resulted in significant weight loss in 68% of the studies reviewed.

Practicing mindfulness is simple. To get started, try spending five minutes each morning sitting comfortably in a calm space and connecting with your senses.

Some studies have found that mindfulness can increase weight loss and promote healthy eating behaviors.

6. Squeeze in Some Exercise

Getting in some physical activity first thing in the morning can help boost weight loss.

One study in 50 overweight women measured the effects of aerobic exercise at different times of the day.

While there was not much difference noted in specific food cravings between those who exercised in the morning versus the afternoon, working out in the morning was associated with a higher level of satiety.

Exercising in the morning may also help keep blood sugar levels steady_throughout the day. Low blood sugar can result in many negative symptoms, including excessive hunger.

One study in 35 people with type 1 diabetes showed that working out in the morning was associated with improved blood sugar control.

However, these studies focused on very specific populations and show an association, rather than causation. More research on the effects of morning exercise in the general population is needed.

Some studies have found that exercising in the morning may be associated with increased satiety and improved blood sugar control.

7. Pack Your Lunch

Making the effort to plan and pack your lunch ahead of time can be a simple way to make better food choices and increase weight loss.

A large study including 40,554 people found that meal planning was associated with better diet quality, more diet variety and a lower risk of obesity.

Another study found that eating home-cooked meals more frequently was associated with improved diet quality and a decreased risk of excess body fat.

In fact, those who ate home-cooked meals at least five times per week were 28% less likely to be overweight than those who only ate home-cooked meals three times or less per week.

Try setting aside a few hours one night a week to plan and prepare your meals so that in the morning you can just grab your lunch and go.

Studies indicate that meal planning and eating home-cooked meals are associated with improved diet quality and a lower risk of obesity.

8. Sleep Longer

Going to bed a bit earlier or setting your alarm clock later to squeeze in some extra sleep may help increase weight loss.

Several studies have found that sleep deprivation may be associated with an increased appetite.

One small study found that sleep restriction increased hunger and cravings, especially for high-carb, high-calorie foods.

Lack of sleep has also been linked to an increase in calorie intake.

In one study, 12 participants consumed an average of 559 more calories after getting just four hours of sleep, compared to when they got a full eight hours.

Establishing a healthy sleep schedule is a critical component of weight loss, along with eating well and exercising. To maximize your results, aim for at least eight hours of sleep per night.

Study indicate show that sleep deprivation may increase appetite and cravings, as well as calorie intake.

9. Switch up Your Commute

While driving may be one of the most convenient ways to get to work, it may not be so great for your waistline.

Research shows that walking, biking or using public transportation may be tied to a lower body weight and reduced risk of weight gain.

One study followed 822 people over four years and found that those who commuted by car tended to gain more weight than non-car commuters.

Similarly, a study including 15,777 people showed that using public transportation or active methods of transport, such as walking or biking, was associated with a significantly lower body mass index and body fat percentage, compared to using private transportation.

Changing up your commute even a few times per week may be a simple way to ramp up weight loss.

Walking, biking and using public transportation have all been associated with less weight gain and lower body weight and body fat, compared to driving to work.

10. Start Tracking Your Intake

Keeping a food diary to track what you eat can be an effective way to help boost weight loss and keep yourself accountable.

One study tracked weight loss in 123 people for one year, and found that completing a food journal was associated with a higher amount of weight loss.

Another study indicated that participants who regularly used a tracking system to self-monitor their diet and exercise lost more weight than those who did not regularly use the tracking system.

Similarly, a study of 220 obese women found that the frequent and consistent use of a self-monitoring tool helped improve long-term weight management.

Try using an app or even just a pen and paper to record what you eat and drink, starting with your first meal of the day.

CHAPTER NINE

*How Intermittent Fasting Can
Help You Lose Weight*

What is intermittent fasting?

Intermittent fasting is an eating pattern during which you refrain from consuming any calories for an extended period of time. Usually, this period lasts between 12 and 40 hours.

Water, coffee, and other calorie-free beverages are allowed during the fast, but no solid foods or calorie-containing drinks are permitted.

For example, if you finish dinner at 7 p.m. Monday, and don't eat again until 7 p.m. Tuesday, you've completed a 24-hour fast. Some people choose to fast from breakfast to breakfast or lunch to lunch. But which time frame works best depends on the individual.

A full 24-hour fast every other day can seem extreme and may be difficult for many people to maintain, so it's often not recommended for beginners. However, you don't have to go all-in right away, and many intermittent fasting routines start with shorter fasting periods.

Here are 5 of the most popular eating patterns for adding intermittent fasting to your diet:

- **Time-restricted eating.** Involves fasting every day for 12 hours or longer and eating in the remaining hours. A popular example is the 16/8 method. It features a daily 16-hour fast and an 8-hour eating window wherein you can fit in 2, 3, or more meals.

- **The 5:2 diet.** The 5:2 diet_involves eating as you normally do 5 days of the week and restricting your calorie intake to 500–600 on the remaining 2 days.
- **Eat, Stop Eat.** Eat Stop Eat_involves a 24-hour fast once or twice per week.
- **Alternate-day fasting.** With alternate-day fasting, the goal is too fast every other day.
- **The Warrior Diet.** The Warrior Diet_was among the first popular diets to include a form of intermittent fasting. It involves eating small amounts of raw fruits and vegetables during the day and eating one large meal at night.

Intermittent fasting is a dietary routine that regularly alternates between periods of eating and fasting. There are many methods of doing so, with many requiring you to fast for 12–40 hours at a time.

There are many ways to lose weight.

One strategy that has become popular recently is called intermittent fasting.

Intermittent fasting is an eating pattern that involves regular, short-term fasts — or periods of minimal or no food consumption.

Most people understand intermittent fasting as a weight loss intervention. Fasting for short periods of time helps people eat fewer calories, which may result in weight loss over time.

However, intermittent fasting may also help modify risk factors for health conditions_like diabetes and cardiovascular disease, such as lowering cholesterol and blood sugar levels.

Choosing your intermittent fasting plan

There are several intermittent fasting methods. The most popular ones include:

- the 16:8 method

- the 5:2 diet
- the Warrior diet
- Eat Stop Eat
- alternate-day fasting (ADF)

All methods can be effective, but figuring out which one works best depends on the individual.

To help you choose the method that fits your lifestyle, here's a breakdown of the pros and cons of each.

The 16/8 method

The 16/8 intermittent fasting plan_is one of the most popular styles of fasting for weight loss.

The plan restricts food consumption and calorie-containing beverages to a set window of 8 hours per day. It requires abstaining from food for the remaining 16 hours of the day.

While other diets can set strict rules and regulations, the 16/8 method is based on a time-restricted feeding (TRF) model and more flexible.

You can select any 8-hour window to consume calories.

Some people opt to skip breakfast and eat from noon to 8 p.m., while others avoid eating late and stick to a 9 a.m. to 5 p.m. schedule.

Limiting the number of hours that you can eat during the day may help you lose weight and lower your blood pressure.

Research indicates that time-restricted feeding patterns such as the 16/8 method may prevent hypertension and reduce the amount of food consumed, leading to weight loss.

A 2016 study found that when combined with resistance training, the 16/8 method helped decreased fat mass and maintain muscle mass in male participants.

A more recent study found that the 16/8 method did not impair gains in muscle or strength in women performing resistance training.

While the 16/8 method can easily fit into any lifestyle, some people may find it challenging to avoid eating for 16 hours straight.

Additionally, eating too many snacks or junk food during your 8-hour window can negate the positive effects associated with 16/8 intermittent fasting.

Be sure to eat a balanced diet comprising fruits, vegetables, whole grains, healthy fats, and protein to maximize the potential health benefits of this diet.

The 5:2 method

The 5:2 diet is a straightforward intermittent fasting plan.

Five days per week, you eat normally and don't restrict calories. Then, on the other two days of the week, you reduce your calorie intake to one-quarter of your daily needs.

For someone who regularly consumes 2,000 calories per day, this would mean reducing their calorie intake to just 500 calories per day, two days per week.

According to a 2018 study Trusted Source, the 5:2 diet is just as effective as daily calorie restriction for weight loss and blood glucose control among those with type 2 diabetes.

Another study found that the 5:2 diet was just as effective as continuous calorie restriction for both weight loss and the prevention of metabolic diseases like heart disease and diabetes.

The 5:2 diet provides flexibility, as you get to pick which days you fast, and there are no rules regarding what or when to eat on full-calorie days.

That said, it's worth mentioning that eating "normally" on full-calorie days does not give you a free pass to eat whatever you want.

Restricting yourself to just 500 calories per day aren't easy, even if it's only for two days per week. Plus, consuming too few calories may make you feel ill or faint.

The 5:2 diet can be effective, but it's not for everyone. Talk to your doctor to see if the 5:2 diet may be right for you.

Eat Stop Eat

Eat Stop Eat_is an unconventional approach to intermittent fasting popularized by Brad Pilon, author of the book "Eat Stop Eat."

This intermittent fasting plan involves identifying one or two non-consecutive days per week during which you abstain from eating, or fast, for a 24-hour period.

During the remaining days of the week, you can eat freely, but it's recommended to eat a well-rounded diet and avoid overconsumption.

The rationale behind a weekly 24-hour fast is that consuming fewer calories will lead to weight loss.

Fasting for up to 24 hours can lead to a metabolic shift that causes your body to use fat as an energy source instead of glucose.

But avoiding food for 24 hours at a time requires a lot of willpower and may lead to binging and overconsumption later on. It may also lead to disordered eating patterns.

More research is needed regarding the Eat Stop Eat diet to determine its potential health benefits and weight loss properties.

Talk to your doctor before trying ETo Eat Stop Eat to see if it may be an effective weight loss solution for you.

Alternate-day fasting

Alternate-day fasting is an intermittent fasting plan with an easy-to-remember structure. On this diet, you fast every other day but can eat whatever you want on the non-fasting days.

Some versions of this diet embrace a "modified" fasting strategy that involves eating around 500 calories on fasting days. However, other versions eliminate calories altogether on fasting days.

Alternate-day fasting has proven weight loss benefits.

A randomized pilot study comparing alternate-day fasting to

a daily caloric restriction in adults with obesity found both methods to be equally effective for weight loss.

Another study found that participants consumed 35% fewer calories and lost an average of 7.7 pounds (3.5 kg) after alternating between 36 hours of fasting and 12 hours of unlimited eating over 4 weeks.

If you really want to maximize weight loss, adding an exercise regime to your life can help.

Research shows that combining alternate-day fasting with endurance exercise may cause twice as much weight loss than simply fasting.

A full fast every other day can be extreme, especially if you're new to fasting. Overeating on non-fasting days can also be tempting.

If you're new to intermittent fasting, ease into alternate-day fasting with a modified fasting plan.

Whether you start with a modified fasting plan or full fast, it's best to maintain a nutritious diet, incorporating high-protein foods and low calorie vegetables to help you feel full.

The Warrior diet

The Warrior Diet is an intermittent fasting plan based on the eating patterns of ancient warriors.

Created in 2001 by Ori Hofmekler, the Warrior Diet is a bit more extreme than the 16:8 method but less restrictive than the Eat Fast Eat method.

It consists of eating very little for 20 hours during the day, and then eating as much food as desired throughout a 4-hour window at night.

The Warrior Diet encourages dieters to consume small amounts of dairy products, hard-boiled eggs, and raw fruits and vegetables, as well as non-calorie fluids during the 20-hour fast period.

After this 20-hour fast, people can essentially eat anything they want for a 4-hour window, but unprocessed, healthy, and organic foods are recommended.

While there's no research on the Warrior Diet specifically, human studies indicate that time-restricted feeding cycles can lead to weight loss.

Time-restricted feeding cycles may have a variety of other health benefits. Studies show that time-restricted feeding cycles can prevent diabetes, slow tumor progression, delay aging, and increase lifespan in rodents.

More research is needed on the Warrior Diet to fully understand its benefits for weight loss.

The Warrior Diet may be difficult to follow, as it restricts substantial calorie consumption to just 4 hours per day. Overconsumption at night is a common challenge.

The Warrior Diet may also lead to disordered eating patterns. If you feel up for the challenge, talk to your doctor to see whether it's right for you.

There are many varieties of intermittent fasting, each with their benefits and challenges. Talk to your doctor to see which option may be right for you.

How intermittent fasting affects your hormones

Intermittent fasting may help you lose weight, but it can also affect your hormones.

That's because body fat is the body's way of storing energy (calories).

When you don't eat anything, your body makes several changes to make its stored energy more accessible.

Examples include changes in nervous system activity, as well as major changes in the levels of various crucial hormones.

Below are two metabolic changes that occur when you fast:

- **Insulin.** Insulin levels increase when you eat, and when you fast, they decrease dramatically. Lower levels of insulin facilitate fat burning.

- **Norepinephrine (noradrenaline).** Your nervous system sends norepinephrine to your fat cells, making them break down body fat into free fatty acids that can be burned for energy.

Interestingly, despite what some proponents of consuming 5–6 meals per day claim, short-term fasting may increase fat burning.

Research shows that alternate-day fasting trials lasting 3–12 weeks, as well as whole-day fasting trials lasting 12–24 weeks, reduce body weight and body fat.

Still, more research is needed to investigate the long-term effects of intermittent fasting.

Another hormone that's altered during a fast is human growth hormone (HGH), levels of which may increase as much as five-fold.

Previously, HGH was believed to help burn fat faster, but new research shows it may signal the brain to conserve energy, potentially making it harder to lose weight.

By activating a small population of agouti-related protein (AgRP) neurons, HGH may indirectly increase appetite and diminish energy metabolism.

Short-term fasting leads to several bodily changes that promote fat burning. Nevertheless, skyrocketing HGH levels may indirectly decrease energy metabolism and combat continued weight loss.

INTERMITTENT FASTING HELPS YOU REDUCE CALORIES AND LOSE WEIGHT

The main reason that intermittent fasting works for weight loss is that it helps you eat fewer calories.

All the different protocols involve skipping meals during the fasting periods.

Unless you compensate by eating much more during the eating periods, you'll be consuming fewer calories.

According to a 2014 review, intermittent fasting reduced body weight by 3–8% over a period of 3–24 weeks.

When examining the rate of weight loss, intermittent fasting may produce weight loss at 0.55 to 1.65 pound1.65 pounds (0.75 kg)

People also experienced a 4–7% reduction in waist circumference, indicating that they lost belly fat.

These results indicate that intermittent fasting can be a useful weight loss tool.

That said, the benefits of intermittent fasting go way beyond weight loss.

It also offers numerous benefits for metabolic health, and it may even help reduce the risk of cardiovascular disease.

Although calorie counting is generally not required when doing intermittent fasting, the weight loss is mostly mediated by an overall reduction in calorie intake.

Studies comparing intermittent fasting and continuous calorie restriction show no difference in weight loss when calories are matched between groups.

> Intermittent fasting is a convenient way to lose weight without counting calories. Many studies indicate that it can help you lose weight and belly fat.

Intermittent fasting may help you maintain muscle mass when dieting

One of the worst side effects of dieting is that your body tends to lose muscle along with fat.

Interestingly, some studies have shown that intermittent fasting may be beneficial for maintaining muscle mass while losing body fat.

A scientific review found that intermittent calorie restriction caused a similar amount of weight loss as continuous calorie restriction — but with a much smaller reduction in muscle mass.

In the calorie restriction studies, 25% of the weight lost was muscle mass, compared with only 10% in the intermittent calorie restriction studies.

However, these studies had some limitations, so take the findings with a grain of salt. More recent studies haven't found any differences in lean mass or muscle mass with intermittent fasting when compared with other types of eating plans.

> While some evidence suggests that intermittent fasting, when compared with standard calorie restriction, could help you hold on to more muscle mass, more recent studies haven't supported the notion.

Intermittent fasting makes healthy eating simpler

For many, one of the main benefits of intermittent fasting is its simplicity.

Rather than counting calories, most intermittent fasting regimes simply require you to tell time.

The best dietary pattern for you is the one you can stick, eventually run. If intermittent fasting makes it easier for you to stick to a healthy diet, it will have obvious benefits for long-term health and weight maintenance.

One of the main benefits of intermittent fasting is that it makes healthy eating simpler. This may make it easier to stick to a healthy diet eventually.

How to succeed with an intermittent fasting protocol

There are several things you need to keep in mind if you want to lose weight with intermittent fasting:

1. **Food quality.** The foods you eat are still important. Try to eat mostly whole, single-ingredient foods.
2. **Calories.** Calories still count. Try to eat normally during the non-fasting periods, not so much that you compensate for the calories you missed when fasting.
3. **Consistency.** Just as with any other weight loss method, you need to stick with it for an extended period if you want it to work.
4. **Patience.** It can take your body some time to adapt to an intermittent fasting protocol. Try to be consistent with your meal schedule, and it'll get easier.

Most of the popular intermittent fasting protocols also recommend exercise, such as strength training. This is significant if you want to burn mostly body fat while maintaining your muscle mass.

In the beginning, calorie counting is generally not required with intermittent fasting. However, if your weight loss stalls, calorie counting can be a useful tool.

With intermittent fasting, you still need to eat healthy and maintain a calorie deficit if you would like to lose weight. Being consistent is crucial, and exercise is important.

Intermittent fasting can be a useful weight loss tool.

Its related weight loss is primarily caused by a reduction in calorie intake, but some of its beneficial effects on hormones may also come into play.

While intermittent fasting is not for everyone, it may be highly beneficial for some people.

CHAPTER TEN

Pros and Cons of 5 Intermittent Fasting Methods

Intermittent fasting for weight loss has been one of the most popular health trends of the past decade. It involves only eating within a specific time window and fasting for the rest. However, it may not be right for everyone.

Some people swear by intermittent fasting, finding that it helps manage their appetite and weight and support their health.

Others may not find this diet a good fit, either for medical reasons or because it doesn't match their picture of a nutritious and sustainable diet.

So, lets takes a closer look at some of the most popular ways to do intermittent fasting, as well as a few pros and cons. The information may help you decide if intermittent fasting is something you want to try for your health and happiness.

WARNING

Intermittent fasting is generally considered safe. However, it is best to use caution when beginning or following the eating routine.

Restricting your calorie intake for an extended period of time could be dangerous for:

- children and adolescents
- people who are pregnant or breastfeeding
- people who have diabetes
- people taking certain medications

- people with a history of eating disorders

Before embarking on intermittent fasting or making any other drastic changes to your diet, consult a trusted healthcare professional to help you get started safely.

3 pros of intermittent fasting

Researchers have already linked numerous health benefits with intermittent fasting and continue to examine them.

Plus, for some people, intermittent fasting fits perfectly into their model of a healthy and sustainable long-term diet.

If you're wondering if intermittent fasting could be right for you, here are a few benefits that might pique your interest.

1. Might support weight loss and improve metabolic health

Two main reasons why people try intermittent fasting are to manage their weight and metabolic health. Metabolic health is a marker of how well the body processes, or metabolizes, energy. It's often measured by blood pressure, blood sugar, and blood fat levels.

Fasting or abstaining from food can create a calorie deficit, meaning that your body has fewer calories than it needs to maintain its current weight. That's why diets that rely on calorie restriction, like fasting, are the hallmark of most weight loss diets.

Research indicates that some types of intermittent fasting can be as effective for weight loss — though not necessarily more effective — as other diets that also rely on limiting your daily calorie intake.

Time-restricted eating routines similar to the 16/8 method are one type of intermittent fasting that has been linked directly with weight loss. Alternate-day fasting and the 5:2 diet may also be effective.

Besides naturally eliminating your calorie intake during the fasting period, intermittent fasting may support weight loss by regulating your appetite to increase feelings of fullness while suppressing feelings of hunger.

The eating pattern has also been linked with other improvements in health, such as:

- lowering blood pressure
- improving blood sugar
- repairing damaged cells
- protecting brain health

2. It can be a sustainable lifestyle change

Intermittent fasting might sound complicated and intimidating, but it can be simple at times. In fact, you might even find that fasting helps simplify your day since you need to plan fewer meals.

What's more, it doesn't typically require calorie counting, watching your macros, eating certain foods that you might not be used to eating, or eliminating certain foods that you otherwise enjoy.

For example, having an early dinner followed by a late breakfast the next day is one way to fast intermittently. If you finish your last meal at 8 p.m. and don't eat until noon the next day, you've technically fasted for 16 hours.

For people who get hungry in the morning and like to eat breakfast, or for those who can't eat until later in the evening due to work schedules and other obligations, this method may be hard to get used to.

However, other people instinctively eat this way already. They may be more prone to trying out an intermittent fasting eating pattern.

3. Works well with a nutritious, whole foods diet

Because intermittent fasting is focused more on when rather than what you eat, it's generally easy to implement with your current diet.

You won't necessarily need to buy any special foods or diverge much from what you typically eat.

If you're already content with the state of your current diet but looking for other ways to continue boosting your overall health, fasting might be something you want to explore.

For example, intermittent fasting might work particularly well for someone who wants to pair it with a resistance training program and a high-protein diet.

Still, this isn't meant to imply that what you eat doesn't matter. There's no doubt that you'll reap the most benefits from intermittent fasting by eating a variety of nutritious foods_and limiting ultra-processed foods during your eating window.

> Intermittent fasting is often used to manage weight and metabolic health. The eating routine might help lower blood pressure, blood sugar, and blood fat levels. For some people, it also works as part of a healthy long-term diet pattern.

3 cons of intermittent fasting

Intermittent fasting is one way to regulate your calorie intake and work toward improving your metabolic health.

Though the eating pattern can certainly be part of a healthy diet, it will likely take some adjusting to in the beginning. Plus, simply put, intermittent fasting is not right for everyone.

Here are a few downsides you could encounter when first trying intermittent fasting.

1. Might go against your intuition

Intermittent fasting requires discipline, restraint, and planning ahead.

For some people, using those tactics to keep your calorie intake within a designated time frame is no problem, but for others, it might feel unnatural at first. This may be especially true if you're used to relying on your intuition to decide when to eat.

Further, if you prefer not to follow a strict schedule, you might find intermittent fasting frustrating.

What's more, if your schedule tends to vary from day to day

because of work, family, or other obligations, keeping your calorie intake to a designated time frame could be challenging.

2. You'll likely feel hungry

Even an 8- or 12-hour fast might feel like a long time when you're not used to fasting.

You may go to bed hungry_several times per week. That may naturally feel unpleasant and unsustainable in the long term.

Plus, at times, it might be necessary to override your natural hunger and fullness cues to not break your fast earlier than planned.

This doesn't mean that fasting isn't a schedule you can get used to. Once you've adjusted to intermittent fasting, you might even find it makes you feel less hungry.

Many people adjust to the routine, and some even find they enjoy it after a few months. Yet, hunger and frustration are certainly something to expect and be aware of initially.

3. The side effects could affect your mood

When you first try intermittent fasting, one of the first things you may notice — aside from feeling more hungry — is ups and downs in your mood.

This is understandable. Besides initially increasing hunger levels, fasting can have side effects, including headaches, constipation, fatigue, sleep disturbances, and more.

What's more, irritability and anxiety are classic symptoms of low blood sugar levels. This is a common bodily response to fasting or restricting calories.

Still, like hunger, your emotional well-being may be another side effect of intermittent fasting that will improve with time and practice.

Once you've had time to adjust, intermittent fasting may even bring you a sense of achievement or pride.

Especially in the beginning, intermittent fasting can have

side effects like hunger, headaches, and fatigue. The combination of low blood sugar levels from fasting and the stress of adjusting to a new routine could affect your mood and mental health, too.

Intermittent fasting_is a weight loss tool that works for some people, but not everyone.

It's not recommended for individuals who once had or currently have an eating disorder. It may also be unsuitable for children, people with underlying health conditions, and people who are pregnant or breastfeeding.

If you decide to try intermittent fasting, remember that just like with any eating pattern, diet quality is key.

To gain the most from intermittent fasting, be sure to eat a variety of nutrient-dense whole foods during your eating window and limit ultra-processed foods.

Furthermore, before embarking on an intermittent fast, be sure to consult a trained healthcare professional to ensure that it's safe for you to do so.

CHAPTER ELEVEN

*8 of the Best Weight Loss
Meal Plans for Men*

A brief look at the best weight loss meal plans for men

- **Top choice:** WW (Weight Watchers)
- **Best meal kit:** **Sun basket**
- **Best prepared meals:** Factor
- **Best plant-forward:** the flexitarian diet
- **Best high protein:** the paleo diet
- **Best low-carb:** the South Beach Diet
- **Best personal coaching:** Jenny Craig
- **Best app:** Noom

With so many different diets out there, finding a safe and effective weight loss meal plan specifically for men can be challenging.

Many plans are difficult to follow, complicated, and time-consuming. Some are even unhealthy or overly restrictive.

Men also have slightly different nutritional needs than women, on average. They may require higher amounts of calories, protein, and fiber per day, depending on factors like their size, age, and activity level.

Furthermore, men are more likely to accumulate visceral fat than women. This is a type of fat stored in the abdominal cavity that may be linked to a higher risk of type 2 diabetes, high blood pressure, and high triglyceride levels.

Fortunately, there are plenty of meal plans that men can follow to promote long-lasting, sustainable weight loss.

The meal plans featured in this article were selected based on the following criteria:

- **Sustainable.** These meal plans are not overly restrictive, and you can follow them for extended periods of time.
- **Effective.** They are based on research and can help support weight loss.
- **Nutritionally balanced.** These meal plans are well rounded and provide all the necessary nutrients.
- **Simple.** All these plans are clear and easy to follow.

It's important to note that although this article focuses on meal plans for men, people of all genders could benefit from them. The one you choose should depend on your personal needs and preferences.

Here are 8 of the best weight loss meal plans for men

1. Best overall: WW (Weight Watchers)

WW, formerly known as Weight Watchers, is one of the most popular weight loss programs on the planet.

It uses a points-based system and assigns foods a certain number of points based on their nutritional value. The program gives users a daily points budget based on their weight, height, and activity level.

Because followers of WW don't have to eliminate any foods, it can be a great option for men looking to lose weight without giving up their favorites.

It can also help promote long-term, sustainable weight loss by encouraging healthy habits and improving your relationship with food.

The service does not sell or deliver food. Instead, the company offers several weight loss support plans, including options with additional support from WW coaches and the WW community.

All plans also include access to the WW app, which includes meal planning tools, guided workouts, and food and activity tracking.

WW is an effective weight loss program that gets you to track the food you eat using a points-based system. The company offers many plans, including coaches and an online community you can turn to for support.

2. Best meal kit: Sunbasket

Sunbasket_provides meal kits_with preportioned ingredients and easy-to-follow recipes for you to make healthy, flavorful meals at home. They're designed to help you save time on cooking.

Sunbasket offers plans for a wide range of eating patterns, including options suitable for low carb, gluten-free, diabetes-friendly, vegetarian, pescatarian, and paleo diets.

You can choose meals from the full menu to create your own custom plan each week.

The service also offers a selection of premade entrées you can simply reheat and enjoy. These could be a great choice for those who are short on time throughout the week.

Plus, you can view detailed nutritional information for each item on the menu. This will help you find low calorie, high protein options to support long-term weight loss.

Sunbasket is a meal kit service that delivers all the preprepared ingredients and recipes you'll need to make healthy meals at home. The service offers meal kits to suit low carb, vegetarian, paleo, and other kinds of diets.

3. Best prepared meals: Factor

Factor_is a meal delivery service that provides a variety of nutritious, fully prepared dishes_that are ready to enjoy in minutes.

You can order bundles with 4–18 meals per week, all of which are individually portioned and delivered fresh.

Items that are low calorie, low carb, high protein, vegetarian, and keto-friendly are labeled on the menu to help you find options that work for you.

You can also order add-on items each week to round out your diet, including snacks, wellness shots, healthy desserts, and protein packs.

Factor provides all subscribers with a free 20-minute nutrition consult. You can also pay for nutrition coaching packages to help you reach your weight loss goals.

> Factor delivers pre prepared meals. You can choose 4–18 meals per week, including low calorie, low carb, high protein, vegetarian, and keto options. It includes a free nutrition consultation and you can purchase coaching packages.

4. Best plant-forward: the flexitarian diet

The flexitarian diet_is a plant-based eating pattern that emphasizes whole, plant-based foods, like fruits, vegetables, whole grains, nuts, seeds, and legumes. It is not linked to a particular company.

Unlike vegan or vegetarian diets, the flexitarian diet doesn't completely eliminate animal products. It allows you to enjoy meat, fish, and poultry in moderation.

This makes it a good option for men looking for a flexible and easy way to increase their intake of nutritious plant-based foods without giving up meat altogether.

Not only can a well-rounded, plant-based diet be beneficial for weight loss, but it may also help protect against chronic conditions, including cancer, heart disease, and type 2 diabetes.

What's more, decreasing your intake of animal products could also reduce your carbon footprint to support sustainability.

"Mostly Plants: 101 Delicious Flexitarian Recipes from the Pollan Family" is one reference book you could follow to start a flexitarian diet.

A flexitarian diet is focused on whole, plant-based foods. You can also include moderate amounts of animal protein, like beef or fish.

5. Best high protein: the paleo diet

The Paleolithic diet or paleo diet_is a high protein, low carb diet that is based on the eating patterns of early humans during the Paleolithic era.

The plan emphasizes nutrient-dense entire foods, including meat, seafood, fruits, and veggies.

On the other hand, the diet does not include artificial sweeteners, processed foods, legumes, dairy, and grains.

The paleo diet is clear-cut, easy to follow, and effective for weight loss, which might be appealing to people who prefer a weight loss program without complicated rules and restrictions.

It's also doesn't require you to purchase pricey meal plans, snacks, or supplements, making it a good choice for those on a budget.

"Practical Paleo" by Diane Sanfilippo is one reference book you could follow to start this diet.

> The paleo diet is a high protein, low carb diet based on whole, nutrient-dense foods. It excludes artificial sweeteners, processed foods, legumes, dairy, and grains. The paleo diet is somewhat restrictive, but simple to follow.

6. Best low carb: the South Beach Diet

The South Beach Diet_is a popular eating plan that is low in carbs but rich in protein and heart-healthy fats.

It's divided into three phases, each of which has its own set of specific guidelines to follow.

However, all three phases limit certain types of alcohol, saturated fats, and foods high in carbs and refined sugar.

The South Beach Diet can be a good option for men seeking a structured program with clear guidelines to kick-start weight loss.

It also provides recommendations for maintaining weight loss once you've reached your goals, which can help ensure long-term success.

You can choose to follow the diet yourself using the guidelines in the book.

However, the company also offers weekly delivery of premade meals, including entrées, snacks, and shakes. These may be a quick and convenient alternative to cooking.

The South Beach Diet is a popular diet plan that takes followers through three phases. It recommends low carb intake and focuses on healthy fats and high protein foods. The South Beach Diet also sells premade meals, snacks, and shakes.

7. Best personal coaching: Jenny Craig

Jenny Craig is a commercial diet plan that provides premade meals and snacks designed to simplify weight loss.

Although many people consider Jenny Craig a weight loss program for women, the company caters to men as well. The service tailors its recommendations to your age, gender (option of male or female), and activity level.

They also offer multiple subscription options, which differ in cost and the number of meals provided.

The highest cost plan, Rapid Results Max, includes personal coaching with á Jenny Craig consultant for individual guidance to help keep you on track toward your goals.

All plans also include access to the Jenny Craig mobile app, which allows you to record your food intake and activity, track your progress, and connect with your consultant.

Jenny Craig sells premade meals and snacks with multiple subscription options. You can use the Jenny Craig mobile app to track your food intake, activity, and progress, and connect with a coach.

8. Best app: Noom

Noom is a virtual health app that can help you make long-lasting changes to your diet and lifestyle to support weight loss and improve overall health.

When you're signing up, Noom collects information about your goals, food preferences, and activity level to create a personalized plan tailored to your needs.

For this reason, it may be a great choice for those hoping to build healthy habits rather than seeking a quick fix for weight loss.

It also provides access to additional support to increase accountability, including a group coach, support group, and goal specialist.

The app also includes resources, such as a recipe library, food log, weight and activity tracker, and educational articles to help you make healthy choices.

Noom is a paid mobile app designed to help you change the psychology behind the way you eat. The service says they help people make lasting changes to lose weight and maintain a healthy weight long term.

How to choose the best meal plan for men

There are several things you should consider when determining which meal plan is right for you.

First of all, consider whether you prefer following a structured program with strict rules and guidelines or an eating plan that offers more flexibility.

Certain plans may also require more time and effort than others and may involve preparing your own meals, measuring portion sizes, or tracking your intake and activity. Consider whether you'll be able to do what it takes to stick with the plan.

If you have any specific dietary restrictions, allergies, or food preferences, be sure to find a meal plan that meets those needs.

Steer clear of meal plans that are overly restrictive or unsustainable because these diets are often more difficult to follow and typically lack important nutrients.

If you have any underlying health conditions or are taking any medications, you should always speak with a healthcare professional before making changes to your diet.

> Decide whether you want a strict or flexible program, and avoid overly restrictive ones. Also, consider how much time and effort you'll be able to commit. Speak with a healthcare professional for advice on what might work best for you.

> There are many meal plans available for men that can help support safe and sustainable weight loss.

For best results, be sure to consider your personal preferences and dietary needs when selecting a meal plan.

Avoid plans that are unsustainable or overly restrictive, and talk with a healthcare professional before making changes to your diet.

CHAPTER TWELVE

"Super foods" is a word often used for nutrient-rich ingredients that confer major health benefits.

Besides promoting overall health, many super foods contain specific compounds, antioxidants, and micro nutrients that may enhance weight loss.

Here are 20 of the best super foods for weight loss, all backed by science.

1. Kale

Kale_is a leafy green vegetable that's well known for its health-promoting properties.

It's a great source of antioxidants and several key nutrients, including manganese and vitamins C and vitamin K.

Kale is also low in calories and high in fiber, a compound that moves slowly through the digestive tract and helps keep you feeling fuller for longer, which may support weight loss.

Try adding kale to your favorite salads, sautéing it with garlic for an easy side dish, or using it to add a pop of color to pasta dishes.

2. Berries

Berries_like strawberries, blueberries, and blackberries are vibrant, flavorful, and highly nutritious.

For example, blueberries are rich in fiber and vitamins C and K

They can also help satisfy your sweet tooth while providing fewer calories than many other high sugar snacks or desserts.

Berries work well in smoothies or as a topping for yogurt or oatmeal. They also make an excellent snack, either on their own or combined with other fruits in a fruit salad.

3. Broccoli

Broccoli is a nutrient-dense super food and an exquisite addition to a healthy weight loss diet.

In particular, broccoli is a great source of fiber and micro nutrients, such as vitamin C, folate, potassium, and manganese.

Multiple studies also show that upping your intake of calciferous vegetables, including broccoli, could help prevent weight gain over time.

Add a bit of garlic, lemon juice, or Parmesan — or all three — to your broccoli for a quick and easy side dish. You can also try adding broccoli to salads, casseroles, quiches, or pasta dishes to ramp up their nutritional value.

4. Chia seeds

Chia seeds are loaded with important nutrients, including omega-3 fatty acids, calcium, magnesium, and manganese.

They're also packed with soluble fiber, which is a type of fiber that absorbs water and forms a gel in the digestive tract.

Research suggests that consuming soluble fiber may be linked to increased weight loss and body fat loss.

Chia seeds are also high in protein, which can help reduce hunger and regulate your appetite.

Try sprinkling chia seeds over your favorite smoothies, yogurts, or oat bowls to enhance the flavor and texture.

5. Eggs

Eggs are versatile, delicious, and simple to prepare. It's easy to see why they're one of the best superfoods for weight loss.

In fact, eggs are packed with a variety of essential vitamins and minerals in each serving, including selenium, vitamin B12, riboflavin, and phosphorus.

Additionally, eggs are brimming with protein, which can help promote feelings of fullness to boost weight loss.

Hard-boiled eggs make a great snack, sprinkled with some salt and pepper or a bit of hot sauce. You can also enjoy eggs in omelets, quiches, breakfast burritos, and stir-fries.

6. Avocado

Avocados_are popular for their unique taste and texture, as well as their impressive nutrient profile.

In particular, avocados high in potassium, folate, and vitamins C and K.

Although avocados are considered a calorie-dense food, they're loaded with fiber and heart-healthy unsaturated fats, which can keep you feeling full between meals to help you lose weight.

Avocados can bring a creamy texture and rich flavor to toast, salads, soups, or scrambled eggs. They also make an excellent addition to sauces and dips like guacamole, hummus, and salsa.

7. Sweet potatoes

Sweet potatoes_are a vibrant, delicious, and nutritious super food.

They're loaded with antioxidants, along with vitamins A and C, manganese, and B vitamins.

What's more, sweet potatoes are high in fiber, which can slow stomach emptying to boost both weight loss and fat loss.

You can bake, mash, boil, or sauté sweet potatoes and enjoy them as a filling snack or side dish.

8. Kimchi and sauerkraut.

Kimchi_is a common ingredient in Korean cuisine. It typically consists of salted, fermented vegetables like cabbage and radish.

Sauerkraut_is the European version of this dish, also typically made with fermented cabbage.

Like other fermented foods, kimchi and sauerkraut are great sources of probiotics. These are a type of beneficial bacteria also found in your gut, and they support several aspects of health.

Interestingly, some studies suggest that probiotic supplements may play a role in weight regulation and affect appetite and feelings of fullness.

To squeeze more probiotics into your diet, try eating kimchi with rice or adding it to stews, grain bowls, or noodle dishes. Sauerkraut goes well in wraps and burgers and alongside sausages, including vegan varieties. It also pairs well with cheese.

There are no rules for how to eat kimchi and sauerkraut, so feel free to experiment with your food pairings. Many people also eat them on their own.

When you're choosing kimchi and sauerkraut, avoid varieties that contain added preservatives or sugar, as well as those that have been pasteurized. Look in the refrigerated section of your grocery store.

You can also easily make your own kimchi or sauerkraut at home.

9. Bell peppers

Furthermore, sometimes referred to as sweet peppers, bell peppers_are a highly nutritious veggie available in a variety of colors.

They're rich in fiber and boast an array of other important nutrients, including vitamin C, vitamin B6, and potassium.

Thanks to their high water content, they're also very low in calories and can replace other ingredients in your diet to decrease your daily calorie intake and support weight loss.

Pair bell peppers with hummus, tzatziki, or yogurt dip for a quick and easy low calorie snack. Alternatively, try dicing them and adding them to soups, salads, or stir-fries to brighten your dishes.

10. Chickpeas

Chickpeas, also known as garbanzo beans, are a type of legume closely related to other types of beans, including kidney beans, black beans, and pinto beans.

Each serving of chickpeas is high in manganese, folate,

phosphorus, and copper.

Chickpeas are also high in fiber and protein, which can slow digestion, regulate your appetite, and promote weight loss.

You can swap chickpeas in for other sources of protein in meals to give any recipe a plant-based twist. You can also bake or roast chickpeas and season them with your favorite spices for a simple snack.

11. Apples

Apples are not only one of the most popular fruits on the planet, but also one of the most nutritious.

Apples are chock-full of antioxidants, plus essential micro nutrients like vitamin C and potassium.

They also contain a specific type of soluble fiber called pectin, which animal studies have shown may help reduce food intake and increase weight loss.

Studies have suggested that including apples in a healthy diet may promote weight loss and improve your overall health.

You can enjoy apples in their whole, raw form for a healthy, high fiber snack. They're also delicious sliced up and paired with peanut butter, cream cheese, or yogurt dip.

12. Spinach

Spinach is a popular leafy green vegetable originally from ancient Persia.

It's low in calories and high in fiber, vitamins C and A, and iron.

What's more, spinach contains thylakoids, which are a type of plant compound that may delay fat digestion and reduce hunger and cravings.

In addition to salads, there are plenty of other creative ways to add spinach to your diet. Try adding it to stir-fries, soups, smoothies, or pasta dishes to bring some extra color and micro nutrients to your meal.

13. Walnuts

Walnuts are a type of tree nut known for containing many healthy nutrients.

Along with being rich in omega-3 fatty acids, walnuts contain a concentrated amount of vitamin E, folate, and copper.

Although they're relatively high in calories, studies indicate that the body absorbs 21% fewer calories from walnuts than expected based on their nutritional value.

Studies have also shown that walnuts may reduce hunger and appetite, which could be beneficial for long-term weight loss.

Walnuts are great for adding a heart-healthy crunch to salads, cereals, oatmeal, or yogurt. You can also season and toast them for a tasty, filling snack.

14. Oats

Oats are a whole grain food and beloved breakfast staple. Their scientific name is *Avena sativa*.

They're a good source of fiber, manganese, phosphorus, copper, and protein.

Thanks to the plentiful protein and fiber in oats, they may be beneficial for weight management and appetite control, according to several studies.

Besides oatmeal, you can also enjoy oats in yogurt, smoothies, oatmeal, or baked goods.

15. Tomatoes

Tomatoes are a tangy, flavorful super food and an excellent addition to a well-rounded weight loss diet.

Tomatoes are also jam-packed with antioxidants, as well as vitamins and minerals, including vitamins C and K and potassium.

Additionally, because of their high water content, tomatoes have a low calorie density, which could help support long-term weight loss.

Tomatoes can add a zip of flavor to salads, wraps, and sandwiches.

You can also use them to whip up delicious soups, sauces, salsas, and jams.

16. Green tea.

Green tea is a potent source of disease-fighting polyphenols and antioxidants.

In particular, green tea is rich in antioxidants like quercetin, chlorogenic acid, and theogallin.

It's also high in epigallocatechin gall ate (EGCG), an antioxidant that may help increase weight loss, boost metabolism, and reduce belly fat when taken in high doses.

You can brew a cup of green tea and enjoy it as is, or try adding a bit of lemon, honey, or ginger for some extra flavor.

17. Salmon

Salmon is a type of fatty fish notable for its impressive nutritional profile.

Salmon not only contains a good amount of heart-healthy omega-3 fatty acids in each serving, but also high amounts of B vitamins, selenium, and potassium.

It's also one of the best sources of protein available, which can help manage your appetite and enhance feelings of fullness.

You can bake, sear, grill, or pan-fry salmon and pair it with your choice of herbs, veggies, and whole grains for a healthy, wholesome meal.

18. Grapefruit

Grapefruit is a popular citrus fruit that's known for its distinct flavor, which can be sour, slightly sweet, and a little bitter.

Each serving of grapefruit contains a good amount of the fiber and vitamin A and C that you need each day.

It's also low in calories, and some older human and animal studies have shown it may increase weight loss and fat burning.

One of the most popular ways to enjoy grapefruit is by sprinkling it with a bit of salt and sugar. You can also add grapefruit to salads, salsas, smoothies, or juices.

19. Yogurt

Yogurt is a dairy product that's high in calcium, vitamin B12, phosphorus, and riboflavin.

Some yogurt varieties, including Greek yogurt, are especially high in protein, which could be beneficial for weight loss.

Certain types also contain probiotics, which may be involved in weight control and appetite regulation.

Multiple studies have shown that eating yogurt is linked to a lower body weight and reduced risk of developing metabolic disease and type 2 diabetes.

Try topping your yogurt with some fresh fruit, nuts, and seeds, or mix it into dips and spreads to give recipes a healthy, high-protein upgrade.

20. Quinoa

Quinoa_is a whole grain super food that has gained popularity recently.

In addition to its rich protein and fiber contents, quinoa contains plenty of manganese, magnesium, folate, and phosphorus.

Plus, it's one of the few plant-based sources of complete protein, meaning that it contains all nine of the essential amino acids your body needs. Its protein content may help decrease hunger and appetite.

You can swap quinoa in for other grains, including rice, couscous, or barley, in your favorite dishes. It also makes a great addition to grain salads, soups, stews, and veggie burgers.

Many super foods can help support your weight loss efforts.

These foods not only contain high amounts of important vitamins and minerals, but also nutrients that may promote weight loss, such as protein and fiber.

To get the best results from eating these foods, enjoy them as part of a healthy, well-rounded diet and pair them with a variety of other nutrient-dense ingredients.

CONCLUSION

In conclusion, obesity is a serious and growing public health concern that affects individuals of all ages and backgrounds. It is caused by a combination of genetic, environmental, and lifestyle factors, and is associated with a number of serious health complications, including diabetes, heart disease, and certain types of cancer. Effective interventions for preventing and treating obesity include a combination of healthy eating, regular physical activity, and behavior change. However, it is important to note that weight management is a complex and challenging process, and requires a multifaceted approach that addresses the individual's unique needs and circumstances.

ABOUT THE AUTHOR

Stephen Wood

Stephen Wood, a certified nutritionist and personal trainer with over 5 years of experience helping individuals achieve their weight loss goals. After overcoming his own struggles with weight, Stephen became passionate about helping others lead healthier, happier lives. With a certificate of Excellence in nutrition and dietetics. Stephen Wood offers a unique perspective and expertise in the field.

In his work, Stephen emphasizes a holistic approach to weight loss, incorporating healthy eating habits, regular exercise, and stress management techniques. His philosophy is that sustainable weight loss requires a long-term commitment to a healthy lifestyle, and he provides practical, actionable advice to help her clients reach their goals.

With Stephen Wood's extensive knowledge and compassionate approach, readers will feel inspired and empowered to achieve their weight loss goals.